2019 年
国家血液安全报告

China's Report on Blood Safety 2019

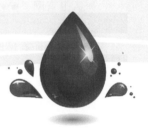

国家卫生健康委员会 编

National Health Commission of the People's Republic of China

人民卫生出版社
·北京·

图书在版编目（CIP）数据

2019 年国家血液安全报告 / 国家卫生健康委员会编
. —北京：人民卫生出版社，2021.10
ISBN 978-7-117-32168-6

Ⅰ. ①2… Ⅱ. ①国… Ⅲ. ①输血 – 卫生管理 – 研究
报告 – 中国 –2019 Ⅳ. ①R457.1

中国版本图书馆 CIP 数据核字（2021）第 197450 号

| 人卫智网 | www.ipmph.com | 医学教育、学术、考试、健康，购书智慧智能综合服务平台 |
| 人卫官网 | www.pmph.com | 人卫官方资讯发布平台 |

本书中所有地图审图号：GS（2021）3684 号

2019 年国家血液安全报告
2019 Nian Guojia Xueye Anquan Baogao

编　　写：国家卫生健康委员会
出版发行：人民卫生出版社（中继线 010-59780011）
地　　址：北京市朝阳区潘家园南里 19 号
邮　　编：100021
E - mail：pmph @ pmph.com
购书热线：010-59787592 010-59787584 010-65264830
印　　刷：三河市潮河印业有限公司
经　　销：新华书店
开　　本：710×1000 1/16 印张：15
字　　数：277 千字
版　　次：2021 年 10 月第 1 版
印　　次：2021 年 11 月第 1 次印刷
标准书号：ISBN 978-7-117-32168-6
定　　价：115.00 元

打击盗版举报电话：010-59787491 E-mail：WQ @ pmph.com
质量问题联系电话：010-59787234 E-mail：zhiliang @ pmph.com

《2019年国家血液安全报告》
编写工作组名单

主编　焦雅辉

主审　郭燕红　邢若齐　李大川

编委　高新强　张　睿　冷婷婷　于功义　王　斐　胡瑞荣
　　　张文宝　马旭东　孟　莉　付文豪　黄　欣

编写组专家　（按姓氏笔画排序）

丁文艺　江苏省血液中心
王　明　福建省血液中心
王兆福　河南省红十字血液中心
王常虹　甘肃省红十字血液中心
王露楠　国家卫生健康委临床检验中心
邓晓林　贵州省血液中心
付涌水　广州血液中心
白　林　山西省血液中心
白连军　中国医学科学院北京协和医院
冯　凌　云南昆明血液中心
朱为刚　深圳市血液中心
刘　江　北京市红十字血液中心
刘　忠　中国医学科学院输血研究所
刘存旭　广西壮族自治区血液中心
刘志刚　上海交通大学医学院附属瑞金医院
刘爱民　中国医学科学院输血研究所
刘嘉馨　中国医学科学院输血研究所
孙　光　黑龙江省血液中心
纪宏文　中国医学科学院阜外医院
李恒新　陕西省血液中心
何　涛　重庆市血液中心
邹峥嵘　上海市血液中心
汪传喜　广州血液中心

汪德清　中国人民解放军总医院
宋秀宇　厦门市中心血站
张荣江　天津市血液中心
张洪斌　乌鲁木齐血液中心
张新童　山东省血液中心
范　刚　上海市血液中心
范文安　安徽省血液管理中心
范为民　江西省血液中心
范亚欣　大连市血液中心
赵　楠　内蒙古自治区血液中心
赵生银　宁夏血液中心
胡　伟　浙江省血液中心
胡晓玉　安徽省血液中心
逄淑涛　青岛市中心血站
徐　红　宁波市中心血站
郭永建　福建省血液中心
宴永和　湖南省血液中心
戚　海　河北省血液中心
符策瑛　海南省血液中心
梁晓华　大连市血液中心
董晓蓉　西藏自治区血液中心
谢杰锋　成都市血液中心
戴苏娜　中国输血协会

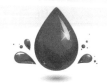

前　言

　　2019 年是我国血液事业稳健发展的一年,我国政府积极推进健康中国建设战略,不断优化血液安全制度建设,提高血液供应和质量安全水平,保障人民健康。以"优化血液管理,改进质量控制,加强安全监测,保障患者安全"为主线,加强法制建设、提升信息管理、强化社会宣传,多措并举,提高服务水平,推动我国血液事业不断发展。

　　我国无偿献血人次和献血量保持持续增长。2019 年,献血率达到每千人口 11.2,较 2018 年增长 0.1。全年采集血液 2 649 万 U,较 2018 年增长 5.7%。

　　2019 年 11 月 4 日,国家卫生健康委、中共中央宣传部、文明委、国家发改委、教育部、财政部、人力资源和社会保障部、住建部、全国总工会、中国红十字会总会、中央军委后勤保障部卫生局 11 部委联合印发《关于进一步促进无偿献血工作健康发展的通知》(下文简称《通知》),就共同促进无偿献血工作持续健康发展提出了新的要求。《通知》在建立多部门工作协调机制,强化无偿献血宣传动员、提升采供血服务水平和健全长效机制等方面作出谋划和布置,要求各级卫生健康行政部门进一步加强血液管理工作的同时,对财政、交通、城建等部门也做出相应部署,为进一步贯彻《中华人民共和国献血法》,建立"政府领导,多部门协作,全社会参与"的工作格局起到重要的保障作用,进一步完善我国无偿献血工作的长效机制,促进采供血工作持续健康发展。

　　我国血液信息化管理水平快速提高。全国血液管理信息系统正式上线,实现全国血站数据信息联网。部分省份建立覆盖全省的血液信息管理系统,实现辖区血站之间联网,部分城市实现血站与医疗机构之间联网等。血液信息管理系统使血液从采集、制备、保存、运输到临床使用全过程更加安全可控。

安徽、贵州、海南、河南、湖南、江苏、江西、上海、天津、浙江、河北等省份依托信息系统逐步建成全省统一的用血费用减免平台，形成"以医疗机构减免为主、网络减免为辅"的无偿献血者及亲属用血费用"一站式"减免的模式。长三角地区血液信息一体化建设、京津冀血液信息联网等区域信息化联网工作逐步开展，在献血者档案共享数据库、用血费用异地减免、血液调剂、不合格献血者屏蔽、稀有血型献血者资源共享等方面发挥重要功能。

采供血服务能力建设不断加强。全国血站从业人员达到 3.63 万人，本科以上学历较 2018 年有所增长，其中本科学历人员增长 1.62%，硕士研究生增长 0.24%；全国血站从业人员中卫生技术人员平均占比 73.43%，其中注册护士人数较 2018 年提高了 1.17%。2019 年，全国血站占地总面积达到 212 万平方米，建筑总面积达到 205 万平方米。固定采血点比 2018 年增加 45 个，增长 3.09%，采血车较 2018 年增加 8 台，增长 0.51%，送血车较 2018 年增加 6 台，增长 0.40%。

"三区三州"血液保障能力不断提高。在各级卫生健康行政部门的高度重视下，"三区三州"血液保障能力得到进一步提升。根据"三区三州"5 家血站调研数据显示，血站建设投入不断加大，2019 年行政拨款总额达到 2 420.5 万元，是 2015 年财政拨款的 6 倍；血液采集能力逐步提高，2019 年"三区三州"血站献血总人次达到 5 005 人次，献血总量达到 8 038U，分别较 2015 年增长 37.8% 和 42.8%；血液成分使用率不断提高，红细胞类成分和血浆类成分分别达到 10 312.3U 和 7 411.5U，较 2015 年分别增长 29.5% 和 35.6%。

医疗机构临床用血管理能力持续提升。2019 年国家卫生健康委印发《临床用血质量控制指标(2019 年版)》(国卫办医函〔2019〕620 号)，从国家层面规范临床输血诊疗行为，促进临床合理用血标准化、同质化发展，提升输血专科规范化服务能力。国家卫生健康委以全国血液安全技术核查工作为抓手，加强对各省血液安全工作的监管。各省级卫生健康行政部门根据国家统一安排，对各省医疗机构进行临床用血督导检查。各省级临床用血质量控制中心充分发挥专业优势，不断规范辖区医疗机构临床用血行为。

(注：本书数据不含我国港澳台地区)

编　者

2021 年 6 月

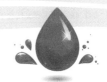

目　录

Contents

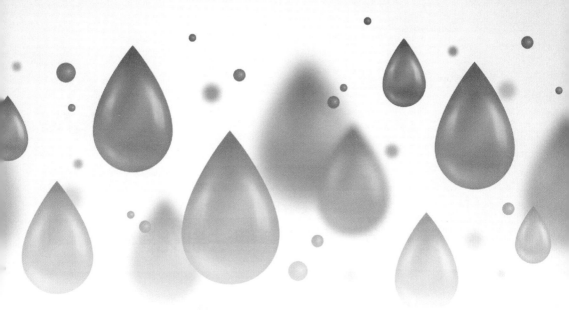

第一篇

血液安全管理

第一章　血液管理法制化建设

一、血液管理法制框架基本形成

1998 年《中华人民共和国献血法》实施以来,我国血液管理法制化建设快速发展,围绕无偿献血、采供血体系建设和能力建设及临床用血等工作,不断完善立法框架,不断更新立法内容。

《血站技术操作规程(2015 版)》自施行以来,对促进血站规范化管理,实现并巩固核酸检测全覆盖,提升血液质量安全水平发挥了重要作用。为不断适应血站技术发展要求,2019 年 4 月 28 日,国家卫生健康委发布《血站技术操作规程(2019 版)》。2019 版规程主要从加强献血者权益保护,完善血液采集技术标准,细化血液成分制备技术要求,调整血液检测有关内容,加强血液储存、发放和运输管理,以及强化质量控制管理等方面进行修订,保留原有体系框架的基础上提高标准、持续完善,这将对进一步提升血站业务工作能力,推动行业发展起到至关重要的作用。

我国血液管理框架逐步完善,形成以《中华人民共和国献血法》为上位法,《血液制品管理条例》《血站管理办法》《医疗机构临床用血管理办法》等法规、规章为主体的法制化体系(表 1-1)。

二、血液技术标准体系逐步完善

血液标准作为采供血相关技术的指导性文件,在血站采供血业务、血液质量和医疗机构临床输血与血液安全等领域发挥着不可替代的重要作用。2001年,国家标准委员会和原卫生部批准发布《献血者健康检查要求》(GB 18467)、

表 1-1 血液管理法律框架

	规划	无偿献血	一般血站	特殊血站	临床用血	单采血浆站
法律		《中华人民共和国献血法》(1998)				
法规		各省、自治区、直辖市颁布的献血法实施细则或办法				《血液制品管理条例》(2016年修订)
规章			《血站管理办法》(2017)	《脐带血造血干细胞库管理办法(试行)》(1999)	《医疗机构临床用血管理办法》(2012)	《单采血浆站管理办法》(2008)
规范性文件	《血站设置规划指导原则》(2013)		《血站基本标准》(2000)《血站质量管理规范》(2006)《血站实验室质量管理规范》(2006)《全面推进血站核酸检测工作实施方案(2013—2015年)》(2013)《血站技术操作规程(2019版)》《关于进一步促进无偿献血工作健康发展的通知》(2019)	《脐带血造血干细胞库技术规范(试行)》(2002)	《临床输血技术规范》(2000)《临床用血质量控制指标(2019年版)》(2019)	《单采血浆站基本标准》(2000)《单采血浆质量管理规范》(2006)《单采血浆站技术操作规程(2011版)》(2011)《关于单采血浆管理有关事项的通知》(2012)《关于促进单采血浆站健康发展的意见》(2016)

《全血及成分血质量要求》(GB 18469)和《输血医学常用术语》(WS/T 2033)
项标准,到 2019 年已经增加到 12 个(表 1-2)。我国不断加快血液标准的建设
进程,努力提高血液标准的前瞻性和指导性,积极开创血液标准工作的新局
面,完善血液标准体系建设,为血液安全和人民健康提供更有力的保障。

表 1-2　血液标准

类型	标准名称
国家标准	《献血者健康检查要求》(GB 18467—2011)
	《全血及成分血质量要求》(GB 18469—2012)
行业标准	《输血医学常用术语》(WS/T 203—2001)
	《献血场所配置要求》(WS/T 401—2012)
	《血液储存要求》(WS 399—2012)
	《血液运输要求》(WS/T 400—2012)
	《全血及成分血质量监测指南》(WS/T 550—2017)
	《献血不良反应分类指南》(WS/T 551—2017)
	《献血相关血管迷走神经反应预防和处置指南》(WS/T 595—2018)
	《内科输血》(WS/T 622—2018)
	《全血和成分血使用》(WS/T 623—2018)
	《输血反应分类》(WS/T 624—2018)

国家卫生健康标准委员会血液标准专业委员会在国家卫生健康委医政医
管局、法规司及国家卫生健康委医疗管理服务指导中心的领导和支持下,有序
落实各项工作任务,积极推动血液团体标准的试点工作,不断推进血液标准体
系建设。

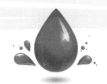

第二章　无偿献血工作机制

一、无偿献血统筹协调机制逐步完善

2019 年 11 月，国家卫生健康委等 11 部门印发《关于进一步促进无偿献血工作健康发展的通知》(国卫办医发〔2019〕21 号)，要求各地进一步健全无偿献血长效机制，做好无偿献血统筹协调工作，进一步巩固政府领导、部门协作、社会广泛参与的无偿献血工作格局。各省(自治区、直辖市)在持续贯彻落实《中华人民共和国献血法》的基础上，进一步强化政府责任，天津、河北、内蒙古、辽宁、江苏、江西、河南、贵州、甘肃等省(自治区、直辖市)均成立省级无偿献血领导小组，由分管副省长任组长主持工作，每年召开 1~2 次会议，部署全省的无偿献血工作。安徽、海南、河南、江苏、江西、辽宁、宁夏、上海、天津、新疆、浙江、河北、云南昆明、四川部分地市等将无偿献血工作纳入精神文明建设，贵州、河南、海南、江苏、辽宁、宁夏、天津、浙江把无偿献血工作纳入政府工作考核目标中。

二、血站服务体系持续加强

1. 从业人员整体素质不断提升

2019 年全国血站从业人员共 3.63 万人(36 307)，比 2018 年减少 0.08 万人，降低 2.16%。本科以上学历较去年均有所增长(图 1-1)，总体增长 1.89 个百分点，本科学历人员增长 1.62%，硕士研究生增长 0.24%，博士研究生增长 0.03%。大专及大专以下学历人员逐年减少，人员整体学历水平不断提高。2019 年全国血站从业人员中卫生技术人员平均占比 73.43%，与 2018 年基本持平(图

1-2),其中注册护士人数较去年提高了 1.17%,执业(助理)医师、检验人员和其他卫生人员比例均较去年有所降低,分别降低了 0.59%、0.39% 和 0.19%。2019 年,血站从业人员中,中级职称和高级职称人员占比不断增加(图 1-3)。其中中级职称占比较去年提高 0.32%,高级职称占比较去年提高 0.49%。

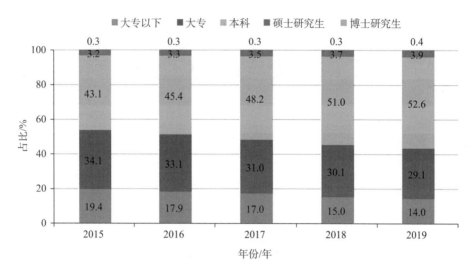

图 1-1   2015—2019 年全国血站工作人员学历占比情况

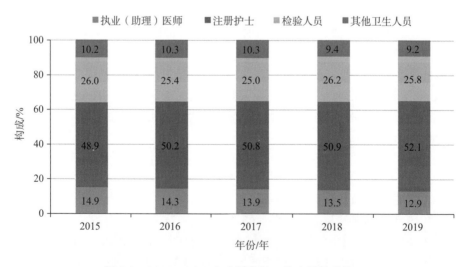

图 1-2   2015—2019 年全国血站工作人员构成情况

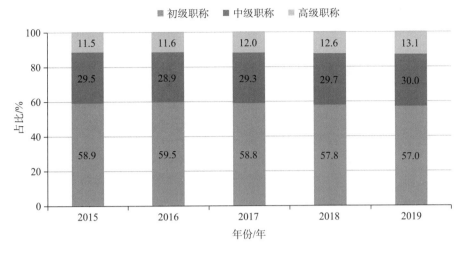

图 1-3　2015—2019 年全国血站工作人员职称占比情况

2. 血站基础设施持续改善

2019 年,全国血站占地总面积 212 万平方米,建筑总面积 205 万平方米,总体规模能够满足血站任务和功能需求(图 1-4)。同时,全国固定采血点、采血车和送血车等基础设施的数量仍然呈增长态势(图 1-5),其中固定采血点比 2018 年增加 45 个,增长 3.09%,采血车较 2018 年增加 8 台,增长 0.51%,送血车较 2018 年增加 6 台,增长 0.40%。

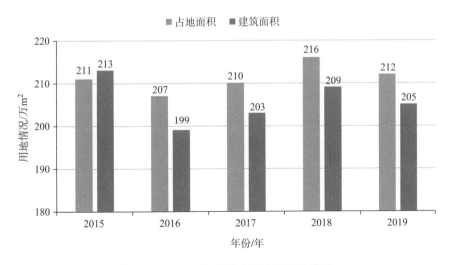

图 1-4　2015—2019 年全国血站用地情况

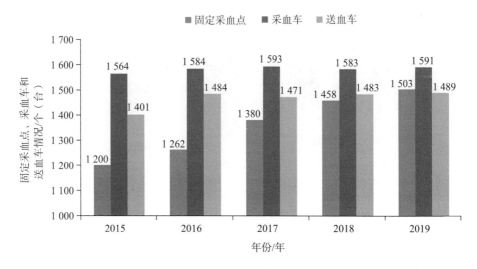

图 1-5　2015—2019 年全国血站固定采血点、采血车和送血车情况

3. 血液管理信息化服务能力有效加强

全国血液管理信息系统正式上线,实时采集全国无偿献血数据。各省血液信息化管理水平也不断提高。全国大部分省份建成覆盖全省的血液管理信息系统,辖区内基本实现血站之间联网,部分城市实现血站与医院之间联网等,使得血液从采集、制备、保存、运输到临床使用全过程更加安全可控。安徽、贵州、海南、河南、湖南、江苏、江西、上海、天津、浙江、河北等省份已陆续建成全省统一的用血费用减免平台,形成"以医疗机构减免为主、网络减免为辅"的无偿献血者及亲属用血费用"一站式"减免的模式。

区域信息化联网工作逐步推进。目前较为成熟的有长三角地区和京津冀地区。为推进长三角地区血液信息一体化建设,2019 年 8 月 16 日,在杭州召开了长三角地区采供血机构献血者间隔期联合屏蔽专项工作启动会,确定了长三角间隔期献血者信息共享联网模式。浙江省血液中心牵头制定信息共享基本数据集和接口规范,确定共享数据内容,目前已完成长三角地区采供血机构间隔期献血者、浙江省不合格献血者信息共享系统建设工作。河北省血液中心作为牵头负责单位,在推进京津冀血液信息联网,建立献血者档案共享数据库,实现用血费用异地减免、血液调剂、不合格献血者屏蔽、稀有血型献血者资源共享等方面发挥重要功能。为推动全国区域性血液信息共享提供实践经验。

三、血液应急保障能力不断增强

2019 年,我国各级卫生健康行政部门在血液应急保障上推陈出新,不断优化血液应急保障预案。四川、贵州、海南、河南、江苏、江西、辽宁、内蒙古、上海、天津、河北等省份制定了血液应急保障机制或预案,安徽、四川、海南、河南、湖南、江苏、辽宁、内蒙古、宁夏、上海、天津、新疆、云南、浙江等省份将应急管理、血液调剂等纳入全省的血液管理信息系统,统一协调、统一管理。其中河北省省政府办公厅印发了《河北省血液应急保障预案》,明确建立健全分级负责、属地管理的血液应急保障体制。各地纷纷建立应急梯队,组建团体献血队伍、成分献血者队伍和稀有血型献血者队伍。各级机关事业单位要组织开展摸底调研,掌握本单位健康适龄人员底数,以自愿为原则,组建无偿献血志愿服务应急队伍,在发生突发事件或出现阶段性血液短缺时,第一时间响应号召,参加无偿献血。山西省与多家单位、团体签订应急献血协议书,对职工进行了体检筛查备案,建立起有效的后备应急移动血库,目前山西省无偿献血应急队伍人数达 1.8 万余人,为临床应急用血提供了有效保障。山东省先后组建全省卫生健康系统爱心血库、血站职工活血库、Rh 阴性稀有血型库三个应急血库和无偿献血志愿者队伍、大学生献血 110 队伍、机采血小板应急队伍等三支应急队伍。开发了全省血液应急调拨系统,强化省内各地区之间的联动,实现血液库存、应急车辆等实时管理。江苏省积极协调民航部门建立绿色通道,确保完成血液调剂任务,完成援藏任务。

四、无偿献血激励机制逐步完善

各地不断创新无偿献血的激励机制。通过法制化建设,加大无偿献血奖励力度,丰富无偿献血奖励形式。江苏、浙江等地在修订地方立法时,率先提出开展“三免”政策,取得良好的社会反响。除此之外,北京尝试引入保险机制,向献血者赠送意外保险;浙江部分地市实施积分落户政策;福建省厦门市将无偿献血纳入“白鹭分”系统,白鹭分较高的市民可享受图书馆免押金借阅、免押金骑行等权益。这些具体措施的实行,有效推动了当地无偿献血工作的持续进步。

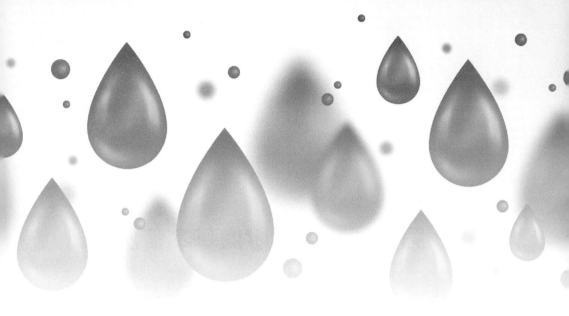

第二篇

无偿献血促进

第一章 无偿献血基本情况

一、无偿献血人次持续增长

我国已基本形成个人自愿无偿献血与团体自愿无偿献血协调发展的无偿献血模式。2019 年,全国个人自愿无偿献血总人次为 1 110.1 万人次,比 2018 年增长 4.0%,其中,个人捐献全血 993.8 万人次,比 2018 年增长 3.1%,个人捐献血小板 116.4 万人次,比 2018 年增长 11.9%(表 2-1)。

表 2-1 2015—2019 年个人自愿无偿献血人次及增长情况

年份	献血 / 万人次	增长率 / %	献全血 / 万人次	增长率 / %	献血小板 / 万人次	增长率 / %
2015	961.3	—	881.9	−1.7	79.4	—
2016	1 013.1	5.4	927.6	5.2	85.5	7.7
2017	1 049.4	3.6	957.0	3.2	92.4	8.1
2018	1 067.6	1.7	963.6	0.7	104.0	12.5
2019	1 110.1	4.0	993.8	3.1	116.4	11.9

2019 年,团体无偿献血所占比例从 2018 年的 27.2% 增长到 27.6%(图 2-1)。

2019 年,全国团体自愿无偿献血人次数为 431.9 万人次,比 2018 年增长 7.2%;献全血人次数为 427.9 万人次,比 2018 年增长 7.2%;献血小板人次数为 4.0 万人次,比 2018 年增长 10.3%(表 2-2)。

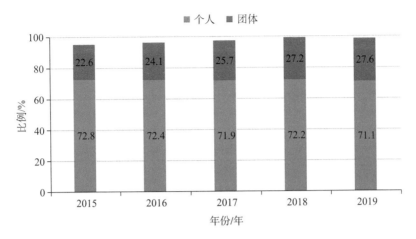

图 2-1　2015—2019 年个人和团体自愿无偿献血所占比例情况

表 2-2　2015—2019 年全国团体自愿无偿献血人次及增长情况

年份	献血 / 万人次	增长率 / %	献全血 / 万人次	增长率 / %	献血小板 / 万人次	增长率 / %
2015	298.5	11.3	296.0	11.3	2.6	3.1
2016	337.2	13.0	334.5	13.0	2.7	4.8
2017	375.2	11.2	372.3	11.3	2.8	5.5
2018	402.7	7.4	399.1	7.2	3.6	25.8
2019	431.9	7.2	427.9	7.2	4.0	10.3

二、无偿献血者性别构成逐步优化

我国无偿献血者的性别构成总体上呈现均衡发展,女性比例呈逐年上升趋势(图 2-2)。2019 年,女性无偿献血者占比为 37.6%,比 2018 年增长 0.5%。无偿献血者性别构成日趋优化。

三、无偿献血者年龄构成均衡发展

无偿献血者的年龄分布主要以 18~45 岁为主。2019 年,全国 18~44 岁无偿献血者所占比例接近 77.0%。2015—2019 年超过 55 周岁的无偿献血者接近 89 万人次(图 2-3)。我国无偿献血人群有年龄增大趋势。

四、无偿献血者学历层次逐步提高

2019 年我国无偿献血者学历层次呈上升态势。无偿献血人群以初中、高

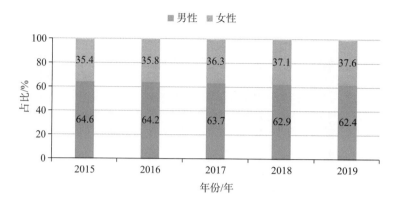

图 2-2   2015—2019 年无偿献血者不同性别占比情况

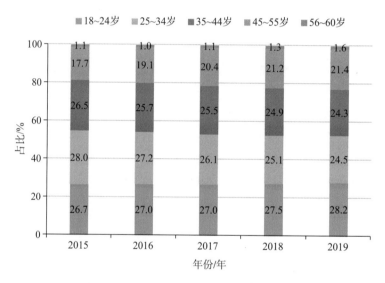

图 2-3   2015—2019 年无偿献血者不同年龄占比情况

中、专科为主,本科学历献血者所占比例由 2018 年的 19.8% 提高到 2019 年的
20.6%,小学、初中、高中献血者比例呈逐年下降趋势(图 2-4)。

五、高校学生献血人次逐年提升

无偿献血者职业涵盖学生、职员、农民、工人、医务人员、公务员、教师、
军人、不明(自由职业)等。2019 年高校学生献血人次占献血总人次比例为
17.0%,比 2018 年增长 0.7 个百分点,呈逐年上升趋势(图 2-5)。下一步应进
一步加强无偿献血招募工作,促进献血人群多样化。

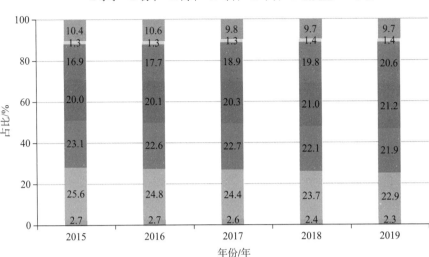

图 2-4　2015—2019 年献血者不同学历占比情况

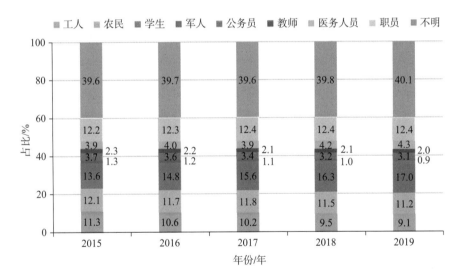

图 2-5　2015—2019 年不同职业无偿献血者占比情况

六、千人口献血率逐年上升

2019 年我国献血率达到每千人口 11.2。在年度趋势上,我国千人口献血率在 2015—2019 年逐年上升,2019 年比 2018 年增长 0.1 个百分点(图 2-6),进一步说明我国血液保障能力逐步增强。

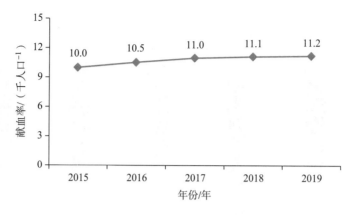

图 2-6　2015—2019 年千人口献血率

七、保密性弃血呈下降趋势

保密性弃血是指献血者主动告之本人存在高危行为,可能影响血液安全,通知血站自己所献血液不能用于临床,血站按规定在确保献血者隐私的情况下,对该血液进行保密性报废的处理。保密性弃血是保证血液安全的有效手段。2019 年全国血站保密性弃血为 3 757.7U,比 2018 年减少了 29.1%(图 2-7)。

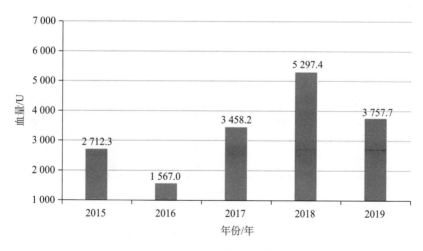

图 2-7　2015—2019 年保密性弃血量

八、 血液筛查不合格率下降

2019 年,全国血液筛查不合格率为 8.8%,比 2018 年减少了 0.2 个百分点(图 2-8)。

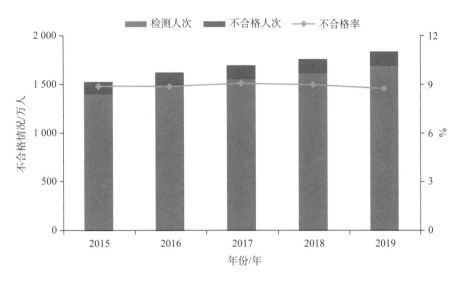

图 2-8　2015—2019 年血液筛查不合格情况

2019 年血液筛查不合格项目主要是谷丙转氨酶（ALT），占比为 54.4%，比 2018 年减少 2.1 个百分点。乙肝表面抗原（HBsAg）不合格占比为 8.5%，比 2018 年减少 1.2%，血红蛋白（Hb）不合格占比为 14.4%，比 2018 年增加 1.5 个百分点（图 2-9）。

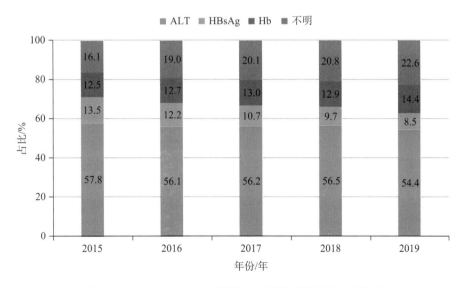

图 2-9　2015—2019 年血液筛查不合格项目及其占比情况

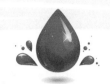

第二章　无偿献血社会氛围

一、无偿献血主题宣传活动丰富多彩

国家卫生健康委员会、中国红十字会总会、中央军委后勤保障部卫生局联合发布第 16 个"世界献血者日"宣传海报，活动的主题是献血和普及安全输血，国家无偿献血宣传员拍摄了以"人人享有安全血液"为主题的 30 秒公益视频广告和平面广告。

各省份围绕主题，利用互联网、电视、广播、微信公众号等媒体平台，举行了丰富多彩的活动，传递社会正能量，向广大无私奉献的献血者表达敬意和感谢。天津市营造献血宣传新态势，新闻媒体组织专门报道力量，拿出固定时段、固定版面随时播出，做到电视有影、电台有声、报刊有文、网站有图、微信有聊、街头有景，打造全方位、立体化、多形式的"无偿献血宣传网"。黑龙江省创立夏季"白衣天使献血月"、秋季"机关事业单位献血月"、冬季"大学生献血季"、元旦春节"团体单位献血期"的献血新模式。上海市组织了全市超 300 位无偿献血者和血液工作者共同拍摄了无偿献血版《我和我的祖国》MV，在学习强国 APP、健康中国微信公众号和市内部分公交车站站牌广告播出。安徽省拍摄了《奋进二十载，大爱热血谱华章》宣传片和《安徽省血液管理信息系统建设与实践》。云南昆明血液中心与省输血协会联合出品云南省首部无偿献血公益微电影《为生命担当》，荣获"第七届亚洲微电影艺术节"优秀作品奖、"第四届健康中国微视频大赛"优秀剧情作品奖。

二、无偿献血表彰活动持续开展

2019年,上海市无偿献血表彰大会于6月13日在上海国际会议中心举行,对本市的全国和上海无偿献血奖项获得者进行了表彰,700余名来自全市各行各业的先进个人和单位代表以及有关单位领导参加了大会。山东联合6部门召开全省无偿献血工作表彰大会,对全省465个单位和31 790名个人进行通报表扬,在全社会宣传弘扬无偿献血的无私奉献精神。

三、无偿献血者临床用血费用直接减免有效落实

国家卫生健康委员会印发《国家卫生健康委办公厅关于开展无偿献血者临床用血费用直接减免工作的通知》(以下简称《通知》),《通知》要求各地要牢固树立"以献血者为中心"的服务理念,全面实现血站与用血医疗机构无偿献血者信息互联互通,实现无偿献血者及其亲属省内就医时用血费用出院直接减免,形成"医院直免为主、网上申请减免为辅"的血费减免服务新模式。北京市、河北省、上海市、江苏省、浙江省、安徽省、江西省、山东省、河南省、湖北省、湖南省、广东省、海南省、四川省和云南省等省份在2020年1月底前全面实现无偿献血者及其亲属在省内医院用血费用直接减免。

河北省印发《河北省卫生健康委关于推进无偿献血者临床用血费用直接减免工作的通知》,对"河北省血费出院即报平台"进行升级改造,进一步简化血费减免程序、精简审核材料、优化工作流程,努力为群众提供更加方便、快捷的血费减免服务。河南省印发《河南省无偿献血者临床用血费用直接减免工作实施方案》,建立以"医疗机构减免为主,网络减免为辅"的区域无偿献血者及其亲属用血费用"一站式"减免模式。广东省建立了统一的信息平台,完成政务云服务器以及突发公共卫生事件医疗救治信息系统数据库改造,率先在广州部分地区启动无偿献血者临床用血费用医院直接减免工作。上海市成立工作小组,制订本市无偿献血者临床用血费用直接减免工作方案,研究无偿献血者免费用血政策执行细则及"直免"资格审核规则,制订资金垫付及转拨规则。

四、无偿献血"三免"政策逐步推广

国内多个省份(河北、海南、江苏、浙江等)已实施"三免"政策。获得国家无偿献血表彰的个人,可以免费游览由政府投资、主办的公园、旅游景区等,到公立医疗机构就诊免交普通门诊诊查费,可免费乘坐城市公共交通工具。

2019年,《海南经济特区无偿献血条例》实施,本条例第十六条规定:在本经济特区无偿献血并获得国家无偿献血奉献奖、国家无偿捐献造血干细胞

奖和国家无偿献血志愿服务终身荣誉奖的个人可以凭相关证件,在本经济特区内享受"三免"政策。河北印发《关于贯彻落实〈河北省实施红十字会法办法〉三免待遇相关条款的通知》、联合省红十字会印发《关于推进落实无偿献血"三免"政策的通知》,着力推动各相关部门落实"三免"政策。

五、无偿献血长效工作机制逐步形成

北京建立了由市区两级卫生健康行政部门、采供血机构和29家主要用血医院参与的信息监测和工作调度机制。山东省政府办公厅牵头,12部门联合建立省级无偿献血联席会议制度,全省17市全部成立无偿献血工作领导小组,及时通报无偿献血工作进展。河南积极协调省文明办,将无偿献血工作纳入《河南省文明单位(标兵)测评体系》。四川联合多个部委,印发《关于建立四川省无偿献血工作厅际联席会议制度的通知》,构建"政府领导、多部门合作、全社会参与"的协调联动机制。

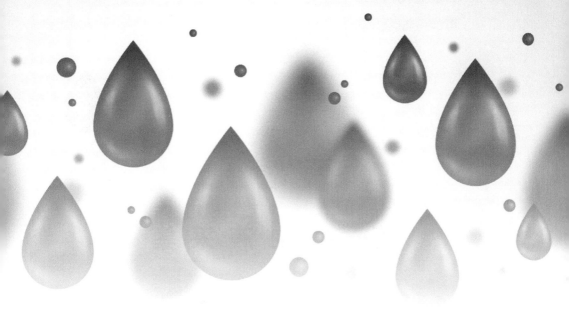

第三篇

血站服务与质量保障

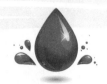

第一章　血液采集

　　1998 年以来，我国无偿献血的献血量逐年攀升，保持 21 年持续增长。2019 年采集血液 1 562.3 万人次，比 2018 年增长 5.6%。其中，采集全血 1 440 万人次，比 2018 年增长 5.1%；采集血小板 122 万人次，比 2018 年增长 12.1%（图 3-1）。

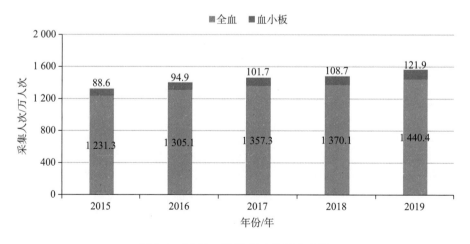

图 3-1　2015—2019 年血液采集人次

　　近五年，全国血液采集总量呈持续上升态势。2019 年采集全血 2 445 万 U，比 2018 年增长 5.0%；采集血小板 204 万治疗量，比 2018 年增长 14.8%（图 3-2）。

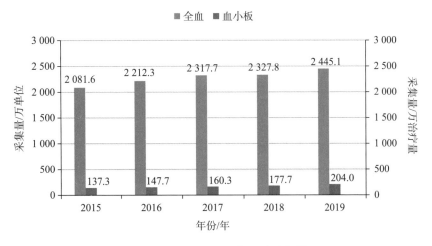

图 3-2 2015—2019 年血液采集量

《中华人民共和国献血法》规定献血者每次献血一般为 200ml,最多不得超过 400ml。随着近几年无偿献血宣传的不断深入,民众对无偿献血的接受度不断增强,献血量为 300ml 和 400ml 的占比持续提升。2019 年 200ml 献血量比例为 18.1%,比 2018 年下降了 0.3 个百分点,平均全血捐献量为 340.6ml,比 2018 年增加了 0.2ml(图 3-3)。

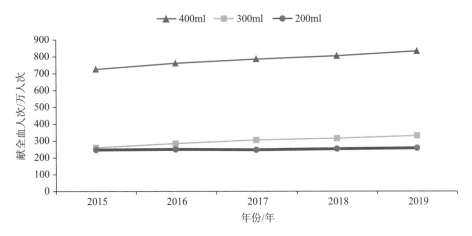

图 3-3 2015—2019 年献全血 200ml/300ml/400ml 人次

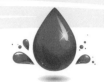

第二章　血液成分制备与供应

成分输血是衡量一个国家、一个地区或者一家医院输血技术水平的重要指标之一。我国自 1998 年颁布《中华人民共和国献血法》以来，输血医学事业不断进步，成分输血比例逐年递增。2019 年我国血站血液成分分离率达到 99.9%。

一、血液成分供应量逐年增加

目前，我国的临床供血主要有以下种类：全血、红细胞类成分、血小板类成分、血浆类成分。

全血：2019 年全国血站发出全血为 3.2 万 U，比 2018 年减少 24.4%（图 3-4）。

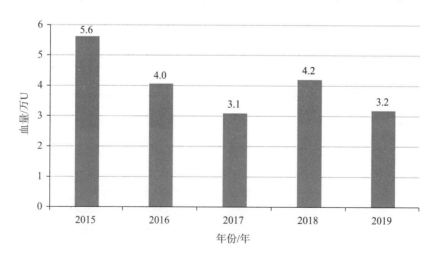

图 3-4　2015—2019 年临床供全血量

红细胞类成分:主要包括红细胞悬液、洗涤红细胞、冰冻解冻去甘油红细胞、去白红细胞和辐照红细胞等。2019 年全国血站供应红细胞类成分 2 447.2 万 U,比 2018 年增长 8.2%。其中,去白红细胞所占比例最大,为 68%,其次是红细胞悬液,为 26.5%(图 3-5)。

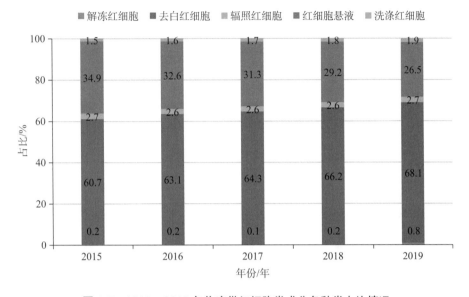

图 3-5　2015—2019 年临床供红细胞类成分各种类占比情况

血小板类成分:包括单采血小板和浓缩血小板。2015—2019 年单采血小板供应量大且逐年增加,2019 年全国血站发出单采血小板 203.9 万 U,比 2018 年增长 14.6%;浓缩血小板供应量较少,2019 年全国血站发出浓缩血小板 50.1 万 U,比 2018 年减少 4.4%(图 3-6)。

血浆类成分:主要包括新鲜冰冻血浆、冰冻血浆和病毒灭活血浆等。2019 年全国血站发出血浆类成分达到 2 422.4 万 U,比 2018 年增加 13.6%(图 3-7)。

血液有形成分利用率是衡量血站血液综合利用和质量管理水平的指标之一。2016 年以来,全国有形成分利用率呈持续上升态势,2019 年我国有形成分利用率为 102.0%,比 2018 年减少 0.1 个百分点(图 3-8)。

二、血液调配促进采供血平衡

长期以来,我国建立实施血液供应联动保障机制,不断完善血液调配程序和库存管理制度,保障重点地区、重要时间节点血液供应。2019 年,我国全年

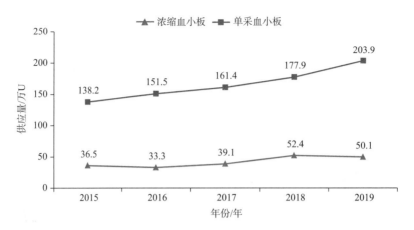

图 3-6 2015—2019 年临床供浓缩血小板量 / 单采血小板量

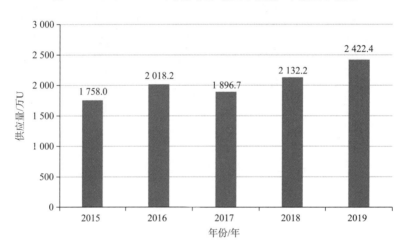

图 3-7 2015—2019 年临床供血浆类成分量

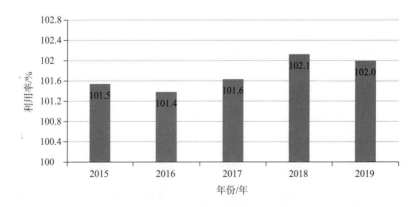

图 3-8 2015—2019 年有形成分利用率

调配血液 314.3 万 U,各地区通过血液调配进一步促进采供血平衡,有力促进血液平稳保障。2015—2019 年血站血液成分库存占比趋于稳定,血液库存基本实现平衡(图 3-9)。

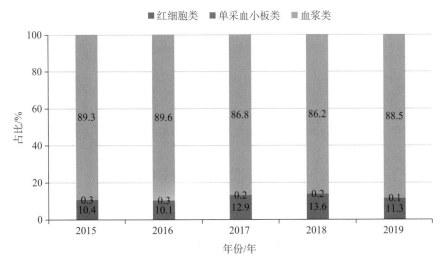

图 3-9 2015—2019 年血液成分平均库存占比情况

三、血液报废管理水平持续提高

血液报废分为检测报废和物理报废 2 种情况。血液检测报废指血液实验室检测不合格的血液报废和保密性弃血),而血液物理报废指因外观原因(乳糜血、血袋破损等)导致的血液报废和超过保质期的血液报废。血液物理报废是衡量血站管理水平的指标之一。

2019 年全国血液物理报废量 174.1 万 U,比 2018 年增加 15.1%;血液物理报废率 3.2%,比 2018 年增加 0.1 个百分点(图 3-10)。

2019 年全国血液物理报废主要是外观原因,占比为 90.4%,比 2018 年减少 6 个百分点(图 3-11)。

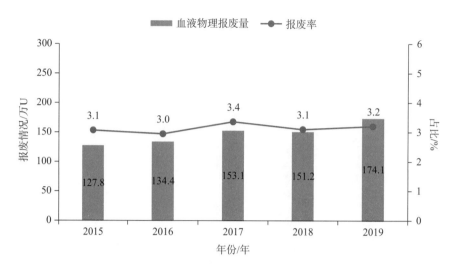

图 3-10　2015—2019 年血液物理报废情况

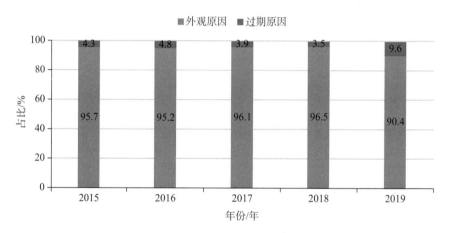

图 3-11　2015—2019 年血液物理报废各类型占比情况

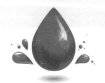

第三章 血液检测

　　血站血液实验室检测主要是输血相关病原体筛查,包括 ALT、HBsAg、丙型肝炎病毒抗体、人类免疫缺陷病毒抗原和抗体、梅毒螺旋体抗体和 HBV、HCV、HIV 核酸检测(NAT)。随着我国采供血机构献血前筛查技术和能力的不断提高,血液实验室检测不合格率呈逐年下降趋势。2019 年,我国血液实验室检测不合格率为 2.1%,与 2018 年基本持平(图 3-12)。

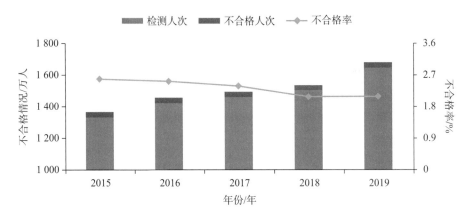

图 3-12　2015—2019 年血站血液实验室检测不合格情况

　　2019 年全国血站血液实验室检测不合格的首位原因是 ALT,占比为44.6%。其次是 HBsAg,占比 19.2%(图 3-13)。

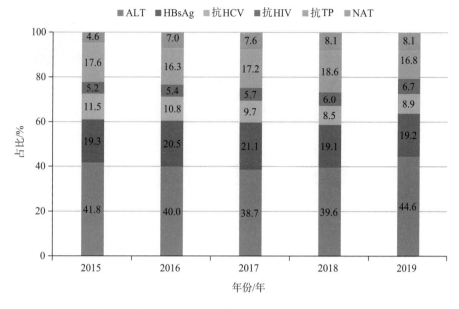

图 3-13　2015—2019 年血站血液实验室检测不合格各项目占比情况

　　从各项目不合格率的年度趋势上看,2019 年 ALT 不合格率略有增长(图 3-14)。

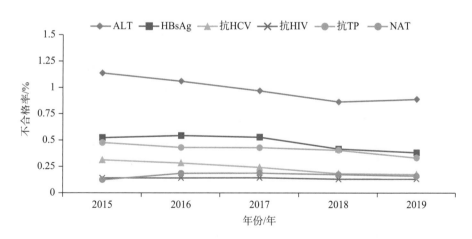

图 3-14　2015—2019 年血站血液实验室检测各项目不合格率

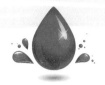

第四章　质　量　评　价

室间质量评价(external quality assessment, EQA),又称外部质量控制,是国际公认的实验室质量管理的重要组成部分。EQA 的基本工作模式是组织者定期向参加实验室发送质量评价样本盘,实验室在规定时间内进行检测并回报结果,组织者分析各实验室检测结果,按照预先规定的评价标准给出质量评价报告。EQA 在对参评实验室进行检测质量评价的同时,还对不同实验室室间结果的可比性和准确性进行总体分析,通过对实验室血液检测能力进行客观系统的评价方式,持续推进各个实验室改进血液检测质量。因此,EQA 是实验室最主要的外部质量控制机制,一直为行政管理部门所重视,在保障血液安全中发挥重要作用。

随着血液检测技术的发展和检测项目的增加,我国采供血机构实验室室间质量评价经历了从无到有、由单一项目到多个项目全覆盖、上报方式从纸质信件到网络上报,最终形成较为完善的室间质量评价体系。目前国家卫生健康委临床检验中心(下称"临检中心")针对采供血机构实验室的室间质量评价包括 4 个质量评价计划的 11 个项目,基本覆盖采供血机构常规检测工作,从而在保障血液安全中发挥作用。每个室间计划包含的项目,因血站、医院、试剂公司和单采血浆站/生物制品厂选择的质量评价计划有所不同。

2019 年全国血站参加临检中心开展实验室室间质量评价的机构数较 2018 年基本持平。部分血库和分站检测职能仅包括血清学检测和血型检测、部分中心血站的核酸检测采取委托方式,各机构参加室间质量评价项目不完全相同(表 3-1)。

表 3-1　全国血站室间质量评价计划基本情况

室间质量评价计划名称	开展检测项目	2018 年	2019 年
		血站 / 家	血站 / 家
感染性疾病血液检测	ALT、HBsAg、anti-HCV、anti-HIV、anti-TP	358	357
血型	ABO 血型、Rh（D）血型	350	348
病毒核酸检测	HBV DNA、HCV RNA、HIV RNA	308	312
HTLV 抗体检测	抗 HTLV	76	81

感染性疾病血液检测项目。2019 年共有 357 家血站检验科参加感染性疾病血液检测质量评价计划。2019 年有 351 家机构的实验室血液检测室间质量评价成绩均合格,合格率为 98.3%。其中 6 家不合格单位不合格原因均为未按时上报。此外,乙肝 HBsAg 的检测性能有明显提高,本年度室间质量评价样本加大了难度,仅 1 家实验室出现了漏检现象,表明技术核查及室间质量评价反馈的问题得到了整体重视,并进行了整改。

核酸检测室间质量评价。所有参加室间质量评价的实验室均合格,即均在 80 分以上。全部正确实验室达到 279 家,占比 90% 以上,较 2018 年有明显提升。

血型检测室间质量评价。2019 年 336 家实验室 2 次检测全部合格,3 家实验室 1 次未按时回报结果,9 家实验室出现检测错误。合计 12 家实验室本年度室间质量评价成绩不合格,其中 3 家不合格原因为未按时上报结果。

2019 年参加血站实验室质量指标比对项目的共有来自 29 个省(自治区、直辖市)的共 206 个机构,其中有 27 个血液中心,179 个中心血站,仅 60%。部分血站存在设备不足、设备维护状态差以及试剂性能不稳定等很难通过室间质量评价反映出来的问题,往往可以通过质量指标的比对发现,因此各血站应该重视实验室质量指标的上报和比对工作。

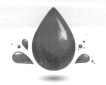

第五章 质量保证

各级卫生行政部门高度重视血液质量安全,加强质量保证体系的建设,对采供血机构和临床用血单位开展血液安全技术核查工作。各地在此基础上,不断强化血液质量管理,通过信息化建设,创新工作模式,保障血液安全。

一、血液安全技术核查不断深入

国家卫生健康委 2019 组织开展了面向 21 个省(自治区、直辖市)的血液安全技术核查工作,检查内容涵盖血液安全相关法律法规、质量管理规范以及技术操作规程,分别对血站、单采血浆站和医疗机构进行现场检查和指导交流。要求各地对检查中发现的问题举一反三,督导整改。进一步提高各级血液质量管理的工作质量,保证了临床用血安全。

二、血液安全执法监督层层落实

各省份以提高血液安全和供应保障能力为重点,通过年度校验对血站和单采血浆站工作情况、换证执业技术评审,确保业务工作及运营情况符合国家相关法律法规要求。同时,省、市、县三级卫生监督综合执法按照国家规定的监督检查频次(省级 1 次、市级 2 次、县级 4 次)定期和不定期对血站、医疗机构和单采血浆站进行监督检查。结合专项督查,推进采供血系统依法和规范执业,完善采供血机构评价制度,针对血液安全重点环节严格检查,及时发现防止血液安全隐患。

三、血液安全防控措施持续优化

各省份定期开展内审和室间质量评价,提升实验室检测能力。不断完善标准和质量控制体系。2019 年,北京完成地方标准《北京市医疗机构临床用血技术规范》的制定,修改制定《北京市医疗机构输血科或血库质量管理检查标准(300 分)》《北京市医疗机构输血科或血库质量控制指标》等质量控制管理文件,进一步强化了临床用血质量控制体系建设。部分省份创新开展远程监控实施日常监督和血液产品的质量抽检,黑龙江省所有单采血浆站全面升级视频监控系统和单采血浆管理系统,实时开展全程远程监控和定期抽查。各省份不断加强采供血从业人员培训。围绕采供血的各个环节,开展形式多样、内容丰富的血液安全培训班。完善血液应急保障预案,对应急事件进行分级,并明确应急保障组织机构与职责,各地适时组织开展应急演练,确保应急事件发生时能迅速作出反应。

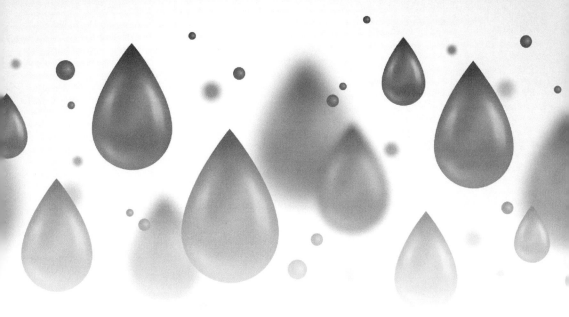

第四篇

临 床 用 血

随着工业化、城镇化、人口老龄化进程加快，我国居民生产生活方式和疾病谱不断发生变化。在《"健康中国 2030"规划纲要》框架下，卫生健康行政部门继续按照"科学发展、统筹协调、公平可及、安全有效"的原则，以"提升依法治理、血液供应、血液安全和合理用血水平"为主线，不断从科学、合理、安全等多个维度加强临床用血的管理。

第一章　临床用血管理

一、临床用血制度建设持续深化

国家卫生健康委 2019 年修订《医疗机构临床用血管理办法》(以下简称《办法》),本次修订取消了原《办法》中有关互助献血的内容,通过发挥医疗机构在健康教育方面的优势,强化无偿献血和临床合理用血宣传教育,进一步增强血液保障能力,保障患者健康权益。同年,国家卫生健康委发布《关于印发临床用血质量控制指标(2019 年版)的通知》(国卫办医函〔2019〕620 号)(以下简称《通知》),《通知》明确了临床用血质量控制的 10 个指标以及指标的定义、计算公式和指标意义,从国家层面加强医疗机构临床用血管理,规范了临床诊疗行为,对临床合理用血标准化、同质化发展,提升输血专业规范化服务能力提出了指导标准。

在省级行政区划内,北京、河北、陕西、甘肃、海南等省份卫生健康行政部门制定或修订了本级辖区内医疗机构输血科或血库的质量控制指标、建设标准;北京、辽宁、河南等省份卫生健康行政部门制定或修订了本级辖区内的医疗机构临床用血技术规范、管理方案、管理指南,从制度上不断规范临床用血的管理。

二、临床用血质量控制不断加强

国家卫生健康委以每年组织的全国血液安全技术核查工作为抓手,加强对各省血液安全工作的监管。各省级卫生健康行政部门在国家血液安全技术核查工作的框架下,对各省医疗机构进行临床用血督导检查,如上海市在医疗机构开展"工作考核",着重于临床用血管理框架,在用血量较小医院开展"模拟输血"检查;着重于实际操作,以区别化的检查,推进不同类型医疗机构的临床用血工作。针对用血量较小(甚至长期未开展输血业务)医院的业务特点,开展以"输注一袋血"为主题,模拟输血前准备、取血与发血、输血操作、输血后续工作等相关环节操作的检查。各级核查、检查工作旨在发现问题并督促整改,促进临床用血工作的健康发展。

在各省级卫生健康行政部门指导下,各省级临床用血质量控制中心充分发挥专业优势,不断规范辖区医疗机构临床用血行为。内蒙古、贵州积极推动各级各类医疗机构成立临床输血管理委员会,二级以上医疗机构单独设立输血科。

三、临床用血培训不断加强

2019年,各省卫生健康行政部门及临床用血质量控制中心举办各种内容、形式的培训班,不断强化临床医务工作者的血液安全、合理用血意识。培训涵盖了临床用血管理、技能、法规等多方面,包括从业人员岗前培训考核、临床用血质量控制中心负责人、输血科主任、输血科技术骨干的专项培训、青年输血沙龙等。部分省份还举办临床输血技能大赛,提高工作人员的专业技术水平。

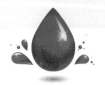

第二章　临床合理用血

据国家卫生健康委医院质量监测系统（hospital quality monitoring system，HQMS）数据显示，部分委属、非委属医院成分输血记录的三级医院住院手术患者10种指征手术院内用血的变化趋势一致。10种指征手术中，剖宫产手术用血在委属医院和非委属医院中无明显差异，心脏外科体外循环手术和腹主动脉瘤手术中非委属医院显著高于委属医院用血（图4-1～图4-3）。

数据显示，在具有用血记录的患者中，绝大多数为异体用血，自体回输占比2.2%。在10种指征手术中，委属医院8种手术自体血用量高于非委属医院。

通过引进使用新技术，医疗机构合理用血管理取得了很好的效果。中国医学科学院阜外医院（以下简称"阜外医院"），采取术前贫血药物治疗，体外循环手术预防应用氨甲环酸，改良体外循环管路减少预充量，采集血标本微量

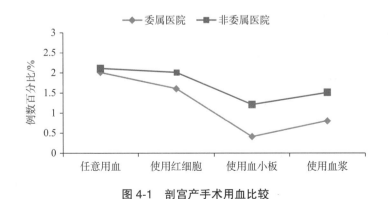

图 4-1　剖宫产手术用血比较

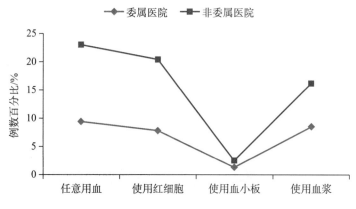

图 4-2　心脏外科体外循环手术用血比较

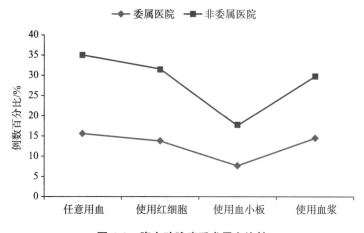

图 4-3　腹主动脉瘤手术用血比较

化减少诊断性失血和应用血栓弹力图指导出血患者治疗等方法。阜外医院自实施多学科血液管理 11 年来,心血管外科手术量增长近 95%,而手术平均红细胞用量下降 68.6%,平均血浆用量下降 80.1%,连续 6 年自体输血量(术中回收式自体输血)超过异体输血量。2019 年,超过七成心血管手术不需要输血,成人心血管手术输血率降至 23.9%,血浆输注率为 12.7%,血小板输注率为 10.5%。同时,术后住院时间、手术死亡率及并发症均显著降低,心脏手术无输血率已达到国际领先地位。阜外医院近 5 年用血情况见图 4-4~ 图 4-8。

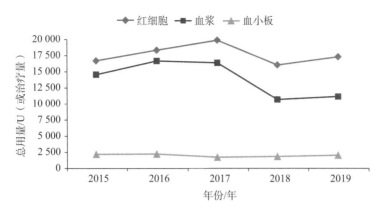

图 4-4 阜外医院近 5 年用血量

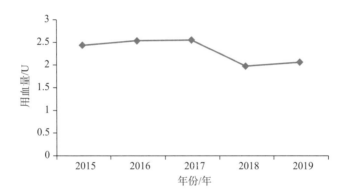

图 4-5 阜外医院近 5 年手术台均用血量

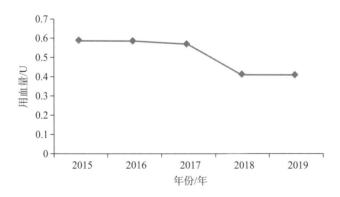

图 4-6 阜外医院近 5 年出院人均用血量

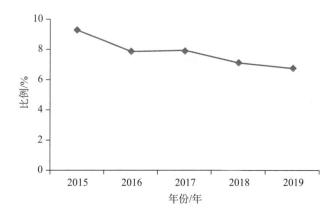

图 4-7　阜外医院近 5 年输血患者比例

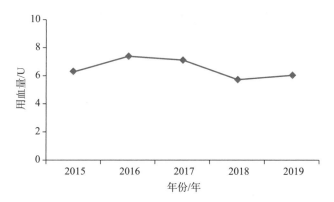

图 4-8　阜外医院近 5 年输血患者人均用血

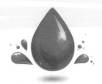

第三章　输血不良反应监测

血液作为一种特殊药品,在挽救患者生命的同时,不可避免地存在发生输血不良反应的问题,而且较普通药物来说,通常输血不良反应发生更频繁也更严重。降低输血不良反应是降低不合理用血、保障患者安全的重要举措。输血不良反应监测是血液安全风险预警的基础,是不断发现问题、解决问题,不断提高国家血液安全水平最有效最经济的手段。因此,国家卫生健康委将"千输血人次输血不良反应上报例数"列入了《临床用血质量控制指标(2019 年版)》当中,引导建立输血不良反应上报制度。

据中国医学科学院输血不良反应重点实验室数据显示,自 2018 年 5 月 1 日输血不良反应数据管理系统正式上线以来,截至 2019 年 12 月 31 日共收到来自全国 29 个省、188 家医院共计 1 933 例的输血不良反应病例报告。

1 933 个病例中,29 例被确认与输血不良反应无关,229 例相关性为可能、疑似或不确定,排除这些病例后 1 675 个病例被确认为确定或很可能与输血不良反应相关。

输血不良反应主要类型有过敏反应,占比为 74.27%;非溶血性发热反应,占比为 23.28%(图 4-9)。

我国输血不良反应涉及的主要血液成分:单采血小板 32.60%、悬浮红细胞 29.97%、血浆 34.69%(图 4-10)。

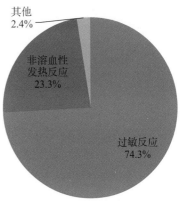

图 4-9　输血不良反应类型

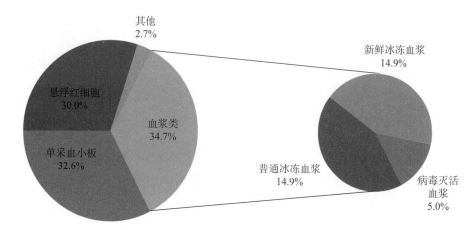

图 4-10 输血不良反应涉及的主要血液成分

94.45% 的过敏反应为不严重,5.55% 为严重不良反应。

2018—2019 年,共累计收到过敏反应病例报告 1 244 例,约占全年输血不良反应病例的 3/4(74.27%)。引发过敏反应涉及的主要血液成分依次为血浆类、单采血小板及悬浮红细胞(图 4-11)。

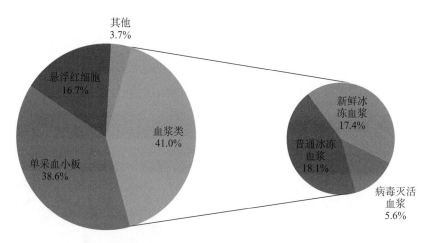

图 4-11 发生过敏反应的血液成分

2018—2019 年,共累计收到非溶血性发热反应病例报告 390 例,是除过敏反应外第 2 大输血不良反应,约占全年输血不良反应病例的 1/4(23.28%)。引发非溶血性发热反应的首要血液成分为悬浮红细胞,共 271 例,其次为单采血小板,共 55 例,血浆类引发的非溶血性发热反应共 60 例(图 4-12)。

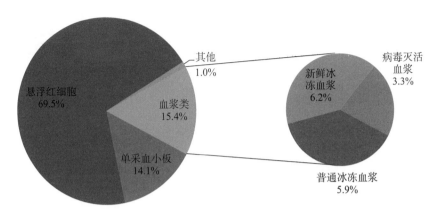

图 4-12 发生非溶血性发热反应的血液成分

自体血引发的输血不良反应仅 1 例,为过敏反应。因此提高自体输血率将有助于减少输血不良反应。

输血不良反应监测是血液安全风险预警的基础,是不断提高血液安全水平的一个有效的工具和手段,越来越受到管理部门和医疗机构的关注。血液安全预警是血液管理系统不可分割的重要组成部分。血液安全预警系统不仅仅是监测输血不良反应,而是通过分析不良反应发生的原因,不断寻找血液安全的短板,并提出解决问题的办法,不断提高血液安全水平。做好输血不良反应监测,及时发现血液安全可能存在的风险和问题,做好预警和防控,防止血液安全风险的发生,是促进临床科学、合理用血,不断提高国家血液安全水平的重要举措。

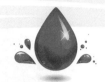

第四章　质　量　评　价

　　输血相容性检测室间质量评价,是国家卫生健康委临床检验中心主要针对医疗机构输血科或血库开展临床输血相容性检测项目的检测能力进行验证、核查和确认的外部质量管理工作。通过室间质量评价可以确定参评实验室的检测能力,发现在检测中存在的问题,提供实验室间检测结果的可比性,不断促进和提高参评实验室的检测水平,在保障临床安全用血工作中起着重要的支撑作用。

　　2019 年开展的室间质量评价项目包括:ABO 正定型、ABO 反定型、RhD 血型、抗体筛检、交叉配血五个检测项目。以上项目均通过了中国合格评定国家认可委员会(CNAS)的 ISO/IEC 17043 能力验证计划提供者认可准则的评审。参加本项目评价的单位主要包括医疗机构输血科、检验科、采供血机构实验室、试剂生产厂商以及部分部队医疗机构输血科、采供血机构。2008 年参评单位仅 200 余家,2008—2014 年为快速增长期,平均增幅为 39%,2015—2019 年参评单位数量增长逐渐趋于平稳,平均每年增幅为 7%。

　　2019 年参评单位数量 2 314 家,包括:三级甲等医院 1 218 家,其中包括地方医院 1 160 家、部队医院 58 家;三级乙等医院 309 家,其中包括地方医院 304 家、部队医院 5 家;二级甲等医院 516 家,其中包括地方医院 511 家、部队医院 5 家;二级乙等医院 51 家,其中包括地方医院 51 家、部队医院 0 家;未填报级别医院 154 家,其中包括地方医院 148 家、部队医院 6 家;其他单位 66 家。全国各省级质量控制部门开展室间质量评价至少有 13 个省份。参评单位约 4 000 家,主要为本省内的二级及以下医疗机构。全国具体参评情况见 2008—2019 年参评实验室数量(图 4-13)。2019 年全国参评单位达

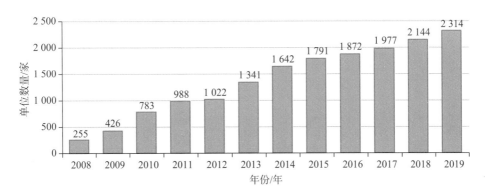

图 4-13 2008—2019 年输血相容性检测室间质量评价参评单位数量
注:以上数据为申请参加室间质量评价数据统计。

到 2 314 家,除台湾省、澳门特别行政区、香港特别行政区以外,覆盖全国其他 31 个省(自治区、直辖市)。2015—2019 年全国参评单位具体分布情况见图 4-14。

输血相容性检测室间质量评价项目每年度开展三个批次的质量评价工作,按照 ABO 正定型、ABO 反定型、RhD 血型、抗体筛检和交叉配血五个项目分别进行评价,2019 年按照参评单位分类统计五项质量评价项目全部合格情况(表 4-1);全国参评单位质量评价成绩为五个室间质量评价项目全部通过为合格,室间质量评价各检测项目质量评价成绩(图 4-15~ 图 4-19)。2015—2019 年全国各省(自治区、直辖市)参评单位的合格率见图 4-20。

表 4-1 参评单位分类统计五项质量评价项目合格情况

参评单位分类	参评单位总数 / 家	五项全部合格单位数 / 家	五项全部合格率 /%
三级甲等	1 218	1 003	82.35
三级乙等	309	230	74.43
二级甲等	516	356	68.99
二级乙等	51	30	58.82
未填报等级	154	113	73.38
其他	66	52	78.79
总计	2 314	1 784	

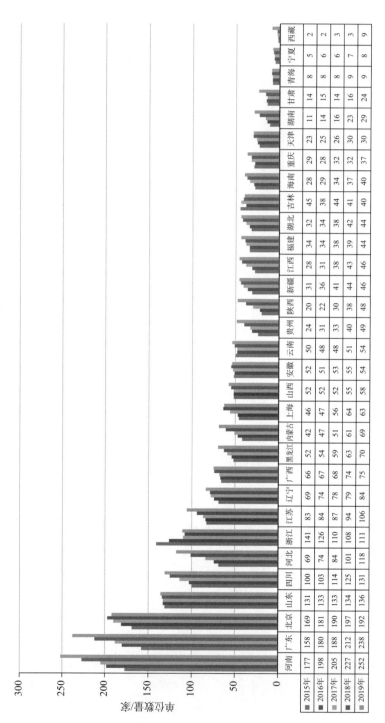

	河南	广东	北京	山东	四川	河北	浙江	江苏	辽宁	广西	黑龙江	内蒙古	上海	山西	安徽	云南	贵州	陕西	新疆	江西	福建	湖北	吉林	海南	重庆	天津	湖南	甘肃	青海	宁夏	西藏
2015年	177	158	169	131	100	69	141	83	69	66	52	42	46	52	52	50	24	20	31	28	34	32	45	28	29	23	11	14	8	5	2
2016年	198	180	181	133	103	74	126	84	74	67	54	47	47	52	51	48	31	22	36	31	34	34	38	29	28	25	14	15	8	6	2
2017年	205	188	190	133	114	84	110	87	78	68	59	51	56	52	53	48	33	30	41	38	38	38	44	34	32	26	16	14	8	6	3
2018年	227	212	197	134	125	101	108	94	79	74	63	61	64	55	55	51	40	38	44	43	39	42	41	37	32	30	23	16	9	7	3
2019年	252	238	192	136	131	118	111	106	84	75	70	69	63	58	54	54	49	48	46	46	44	44	40	40	37	30	29	24	9	8	9

图 4-14　2015—2019 年全国各省省份参评分布情况

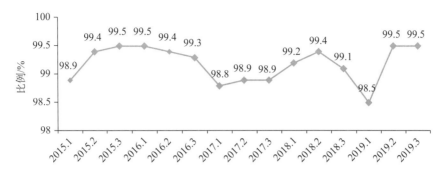

图 4-15 2015—2019 年 ABO 正定型检测项目质量评价成绩
注:2015.1 表示是 2015 年第一批次室间质量评价,其他依此类推。

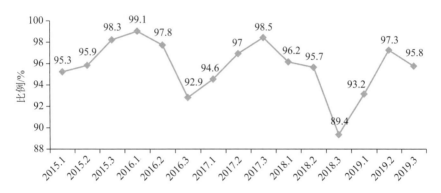

图 4-16 2015—2019 年 ABO 反定型检测项目质量评价成绩
注:2015.1 表示是 2015 年第一批次室间质量评价,其他依此类推。

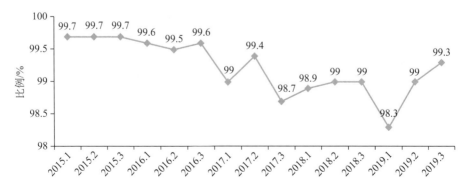

图 4-17 2015—2019 年 RhD 血型检测项目质量评价成绩
注:2015.1 表示是 2015 年第一批次室间质量评价,其他依此类推。

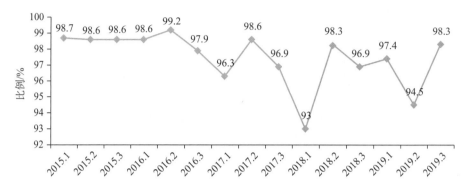

图 4-18 2015—2019 年抗体筛检检测项目质量评价成绩

注:2015.1 表示是 2015 年第一批次室间质量评价,其他依此类推。

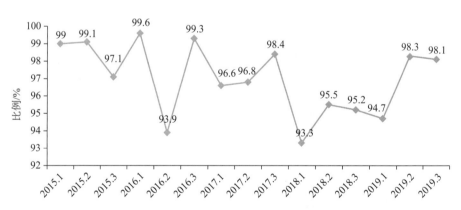

图 4-19 2015—2019 年交叉配血检测项目质量评价成绩

注:2015.1 表示是 2015 年第一批次室间质量评价,其他依此类推。

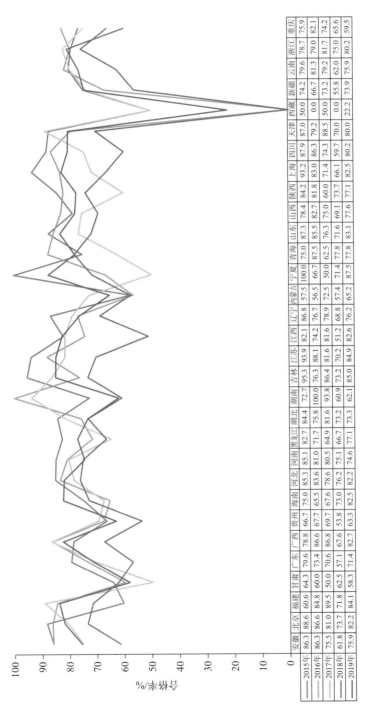

	安徽	北京	福建	甘肃	广东	广西	贵州	海南	河北	河南	黑龙江	湖北	湖南	吉林	江苏	江西	辽宁	内蒙古	宁夏	青海	山东	山西	陕西	上海	四川	天津	西藏	新疆	云南	浙江	重庆
2015年	86.3	88.6	60.6	64.3	79.6	78.8	66.7	75.0	85.3	85.1	82.7	84.4	72.7	95.3	93.9	82.1	86.8	57.5	100.0	75.0	87.3	78.4	84.2	93.2	87.9	87.0	50.0	74.2	79.6	78.7	75.9
2016年	86.3	86.6	84.8	60.0	73.4	86.6	67.7	65.5	83.6	81.0	71.7	75.8	100.0	76.3	88.1	74.2	76.7	56.5	66.7	87.5	85.5	82.7	81.8	83.0	86.3	79.2	0.0	66.7	81.3	79.0	82.1
2017年	75.5	81.0	89.5	50.0	70.6	86.8	69.7	67.6	78.6	80.5	64.9	81.6	93.8	86.4	81.6	81.6	78.9	72.5	50.0	62.5	76.3	75.0	60.0	71.4	74.3	88.5	50.0	73.2	79.2	81.7	74.2
2018年	61.8	73.7	71.8	62.5	57.1	67.6	53.8	73.0	76.2	75.1	66.7	73.2	60.9	73.2	70.2	51.2	68.8	57.4	71.4	77.8	71.6	69.1	73.7	66.1	59.7	70.0	0.0	55.8	62.0	75.0	65.6
2019年	75.9	82.2	84.1	58.3	71.4	82.7	63.3	82.5	82.2	74.6	77.1	73.3	62.1	85.0	84.9	82.6	76.2	65.2	87.5	77.8	83.1	77.6	77.1	82.5	80.2	80.0	22.2	73.9	75.9	80.2	59.5

图 4-20 2015—2019 年全国各省份参评单位全部五项合格率

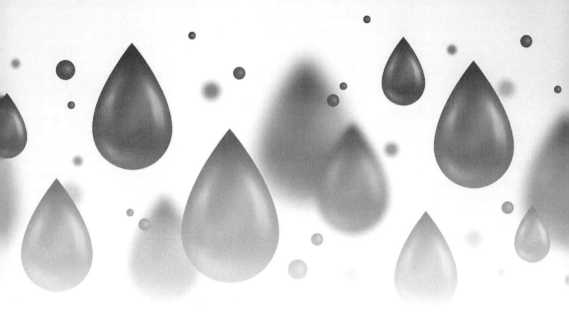

第五篇

单 采 血 浆

第一章　浆站建设与发展

一、浆站数量持续增加

2019 年我国有 26 个省（自治区、直辖市）和新疆生产建设兵团单采血浆站，其中新疆生产建设兵团首次设置浆站。全国单采血浆站总数从 2015 年 182 个增加至 237 个，四川、广东和广西三省份的单采血浆站数量占全国总数的 36.3%（图 5-1）。

二、浆站信息化建设持续增强

2019 年，浙江省研发完成单采血浆站数据采集与报送系统，该省血液中心牵头制定信息共享基本数据集和接口规范，确定共享的数据内容，目前已完成全省不合格献血者与不合格献血浆者信息共享系统建设工作。山西省印发了《山西省血液管理信息系统建设实施方案》，各单采血浆站信息管理系统执行全省统一的编码标准和流程控制体系，与省级血液管理信息系统平台实现数据对接。甘肃省单采浆站监管平台已搭建完成，浆站监管将迈入信息化轨道。

调查结果显示，2019 年 19 家血液制品企业在设的 169 个单采血浆站共投入了 2 427.1 万元用于信息化系统的更换或升级。

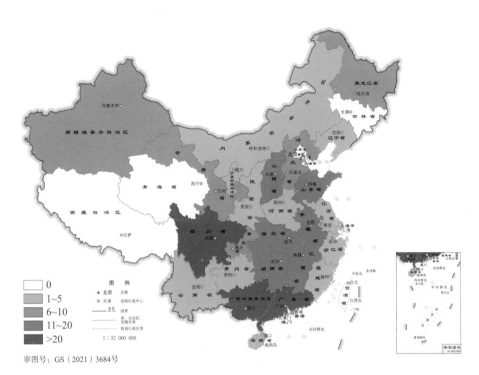

图 5-1　2019 年全国单采血浆站区域分布示意图
（注：本图数据不含我国港澳台地区）

审图号：GS（2021）3684号

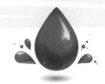

第二章　献血浆者和血浆采集

一、献血浆者

全国在册合格献血浆者人数为366.7万人。其中,职业分布以农民为主,占比 75%(图 5-2);其次为其他职业,占比 17%。2019 年,根据各省(自治区和新疆生产建设兵团)报送数据,我国采集原料血浆总量较上一年增长 13.6%。其中 17 个省(自治区、直辖市和新疆生产建设兵团)较上一年度出现增长。全国献血浆人次数为 2 565.4 万人次。原料血浆采集量最大的是四川省,其次是山东省和广西壮族自治区。

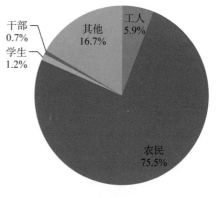

图 5-2　2019 年合格献血浆者不同职业占比情况

二、献血浆者服务不断加强

调查结果显示,19 家血液制品企业共投入 35 748 万元用于献血浆者服务改善。包括制定浆站标准化服务规范、编写印制《采供血机构工作人员文明服务手册》、改造浆站基础硬件设施、提高献血浆者献浆环境舒适度、给予献血浆者及家属使用企业生产的血液制品的折扣优惠、每年不定期对献血浆者进行走访慰问、联合政府到献浆员所在地开展健康扶贫活动,对申请困难补助的献血浆者发放补助等。

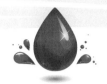

第三章　血　浆　检　测

一、浆站实验室检测

单采血浆站按照国家要求对原料血浆开展实验室检测。主要检测项目包括 ALT、HBsAg、丙型肝炎病毒抗体(抗 HCV)、人类免疫缺陷病毒抗体(抗 HIV)和梅毒螺旋体抗体(抗 TP)。

2019 年,全国单采血浆站实验室检测不合格总数为 3.3 万份。其中 HBsAg 检测不合格数最高,占比 53%(图 5-3);其次为 ALT 检测不合格,占比 25%。

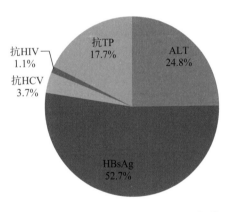

图 5-3　2019 年全国单采血浆站血浆检测不合格情况

二、实验室室间质量评价

2019 年参加感染性疾病血液检测质量评价计划的单采血浆站有 52 个,较 2018 年增加 6 个。52 家单采血浆站实验室血液检测室间质量评价成绩均合格,合格率为 100%。2019 年报名参加质量评价计划的单采血浆站为 117 家,较 2018 年翻一番(图 5-4)。

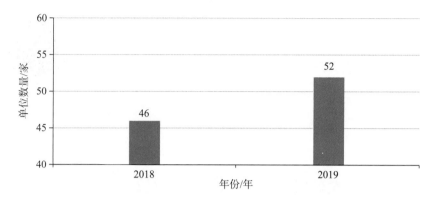

图 5-4　2018—2019 年室间质量评价项目单采血浆站 / 生物制品厂参评单位数

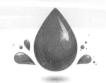

第四章　质量管理与监督

　　各级政府高度重视单采血浆站质量管理和监督。各省卫生健康行政部门不断加强本省单采血浆站的监管,组织核查小组针对浆站开展督导检查,督促整改。

　　部分省级卫生健康部门制定出台地方性浆站规范化文件。江西省组织制定《江西省单采血浆站不良执业行为记分管理办法(征求意见稿)》和《江西省单采血浆站现场检查评估标准(征求意见稿)》,拟于 2020 年实施。广东省起草《单采血浆站行政审批工作指引》《关于全面加强全省单采血浆站管理工作的通知》和《广东省单采血浆机构不良执业行为记分管理办法(试行)》,健全单采血浆站管理制度。

　　浙江省、安徽省、湖南省、陕西省等依托省级血液管理信息系统平台,对浆站进行远程实时管理,单采血浆站质量管理水平进一步提高。

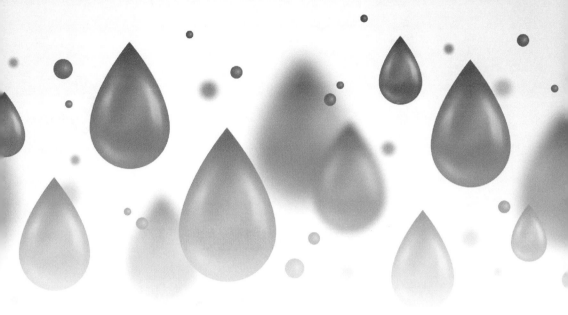

第六篇

输血医学科研与教育

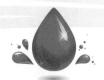

第一章　输血医学科研

一、科研人才队伍建设

2019 年,经过对全国 19 个省级血液中心、2 个计划单列市(大连、青岛)和部分研究所的调查统计,大多数省级血液中心均设置了专职科研人员。在专职科研人员中,本科学历占比最大,约为 44%,本科及其以上学历占比约为 92%,研究生占比约为 36%,博士及博士后占比约为 12%(图 6-1)。在专职科研人员中,中级及其以上职称占比约为 75%,其中正高占比为 16%,副高占比为 23%(图 6-2)。

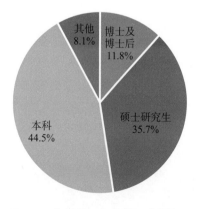

图 6-1　专职科研人员学历分布情况

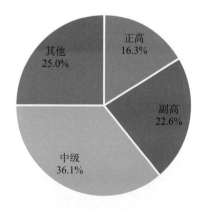

图 6-2　专职科研人员职称分布情况

二、科研项目

据不完全统计,2019 年获批国家级科研项目共计 6 项,经费约 134 万元,其中中国医学科学院输血研究所、上海市血液中心、成都市血液中心和浙江省血液中心获批国家自然科学基金项目。乌鲁木齐市血液中心的 HBV 献血者的随访研究项目获得国家卫生健康委青年科技计划项目。省部级科研项目共计 35 项,经费共计 569 万元,研究内容涵盖干细胞、临床输血、决策模型研究、人才教育和机构建设和输血传播疾病等领域。国家级在研项目共 12 个,总经费共计 800 余万元,主要集中在中国医学科学院输血研究所、上海市血液中心、浙江省血液中心和新疆医科大学第六附属医院等。省部级在研项目共 43 个,总经费共计约 700 万元(图 6-3)。

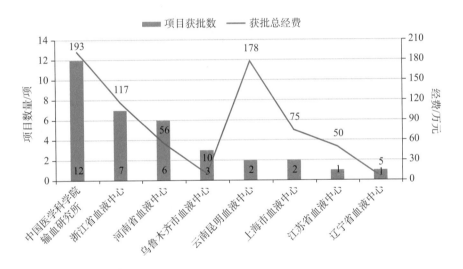

图 6-3　2019 年省部级以上项目获批总经费单位前八名排名

三、科技成果

据不完全统计,2019 年获得国家级、省部级、市(州)及科技奖励 6 项,其中云南九个少数民族 KIR 及其 HLA 配体基因多态性研究项目由云南昆明血液中心和中国医学科学院输血研究所联合获得 2 项科技奖,剩下 4 项获奖单位分别是中国医学科学院、甘肃省红十字血液中心、大连市血液中心和青岛市中心血站。获授权国家发明专利 12 项,实用新型专利 35 项,其中发明专利包括人血小板血型的多重 PCR 检测方法及试剂盒、采血管自动烘干机、IVIG 中 IgG Fab 片段和 Fc 片段唾液酸含量的测定方法和抗血小板黏附且不影响血小

板功能的聚酯材料的制备方法等。青岛市中心血站获批国家发明专利 7 项,
实用新型专利 30 项,其内容涵盖采血装置、溶液稀释装置、采血袋、检验检测
方法等领域(图 6-4~图 6-6)。

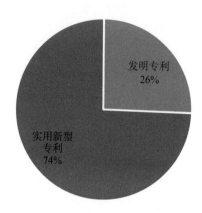

图 6-4　获批专利类别情况

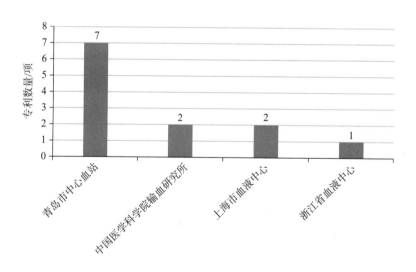

图 6-5　2019 年获批国家发明专利情况

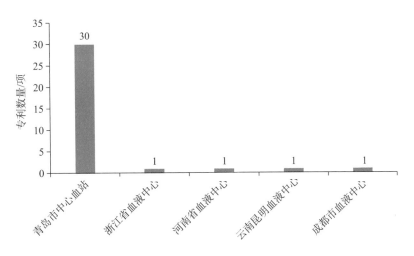

图 6-6 2019 年获批实用新型专利情况

四、科研论文

据不完全统计,2019 年,输血行业单位为第一作者或第一通信作者发表的 SCI 论文共计 80 篇,其中中国医学科学院输血研究所发表篇数最多,达 19篇,累计影响因子总数为 55.89;其次是浙江省血液中心发表 18 篇,累计影响因子总数 50.4;上海市血液中心发表 12 篇,累计影响因子总数 39。论文内容包括免疫血液学研究、经输血传染性疾病病原体及其检测研究和生物化学等领域。中文核心共计发表 107 篇,非中文核心期刊共计 239 篇(图 6-7~图 6-9)。

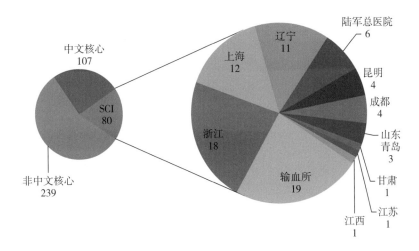

图 6-7 2019 年输血行业 SCI 文章发表情况

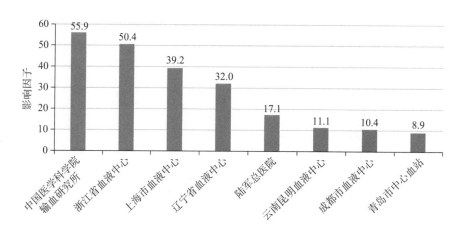

图 6-8　SCI 文章发表总影响因子前 8 名单位

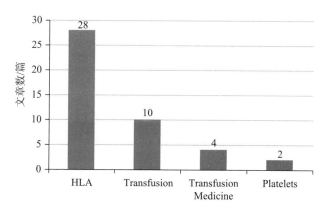

图 6-9　发表 SCI 文章总数前 4 位学术期刊

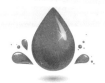

第二章 输血医学教育

近年来,各采供血机构和临床用血医疗机构持续加强继续教育管理培训,设置专门机构负责,完善员工参加继续医学教育制度,制定培训计划。员工职称晋升与每年所获继教学分挂钩。2019年,举办各类国家级、省级继续医学教育项目共计53次,学员数量累计5 740人次,超过1 100学时。教学内容覆盖实验室生物安全与管理、无偿献血宣传招募、临床输血管理和血液检测等领域。

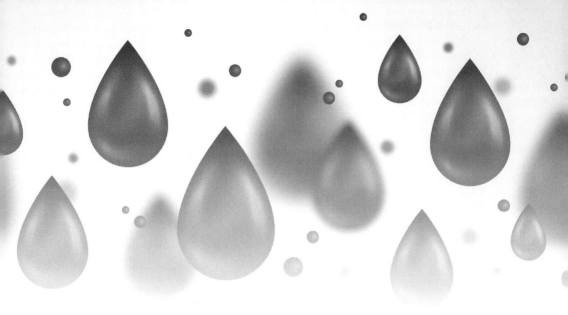

第七篇

"三区三州"采供血事业发展

"三区三州"的"三区"是指西藏自治区和青海、四川、甘肃、云南四省藏区及南疆的和田地区、阿克苏地区、喀什地区、克孜勒苏柯尔克孜自治州四地区;"三州"是指四川凉山州、云南怒江州、甘肃临夏州。"三区三州"是国家层面的深度贫困地区。近年来,在各级卫生健康行政部门的高度重视下,"三区三州"的血液保障能力不断提高。

一、血站服务体系基本健全

"三区三州"血站建设投入不断增加,服务体系不断完善,2019 年"三区三州"已建设 24 家血站。根据调研"三区三州"5 家血站反馈数据显示(表 7-1),此 5 家血站 2019 年财政拨款总额为 2 420.5 万元,是 2015 年财政拨款的 6 倍(图 7-1)。

表 7-1 "三区三州"部分血站基本情况

省份	单位名称	人员编制数 / 名	实际在岗人员 / 名	用房面积 /m²
青海	玉树州中心血站	8	8	1 000
青海	果洛州中心血站	8	7	960
青海	海北州中心血站	11	11	634
新疆	克孜勒苏柯尔克孜自治州中心血站	15	13	—
四川	甘孜州中心血站	20	13	1 084

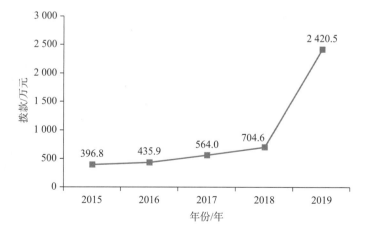

图 7-1 2019 年"三区三州"部分血站财政拨款情况

二、血液采集能力逐步提高

2019 年,5 家血站献血总人次为 5 005 人次,献血总量 8 038U,较 2015 年分别增长 37.8% 和 42.8%(图 7-2)。其中,个人自愿无偿献血比例为 89.6%(图 7-3)。供血医院总数从 31 个增长至 40 个,最远供血距离从 1 152 公里增长至 1 199.1 公里(图 7-4)。

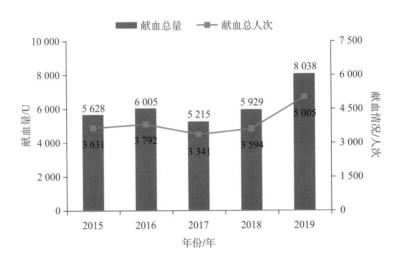

图 7-2 2015—2019 年"三区三州"部分血站献血情况

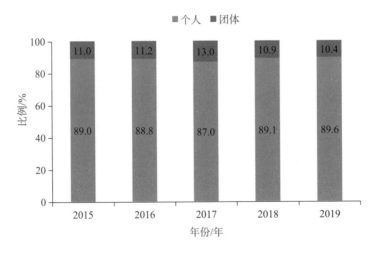

图 7-3 2015—2019 年"三区三州"部分血站个人和团体自愿无偿献血所占比例情况

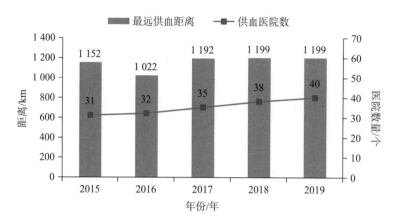

图 7-4　2015—2019 年"三区三州"部分血站供血医院情况

三、血液供应能力不断加强

目前,5 家血站临床供血种类主要有全血、红细胞类成分和血浆类成分,以红细胞类成分占比最高。其中,2019 年供应全血仅 20.1U,较 2015 年减少 84.9%;红细胞类成分和血浆类成分 2019 年分别发出 10 312.3U 和 7 411.5U,较 2015 年分别增长 29.5% 和 35.6%(图 7-5)。

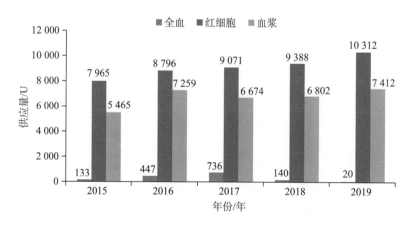

图 7-5　2015—2019 年"三区三州"部分血站临床供应血液情况

四、血液检测

2015—2019 年,5 家血站献血前血液检测不合格率略有上升,从 6.1% 增加至 6.8%;采集后血液实验室检测不合格率从 5.0% 下降至 3.7%,最后上升至 6.4%(图 7-6)。

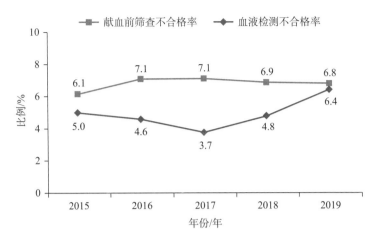

图 7-6 2015—2019 年"三区三州"部分血站血液检测情况

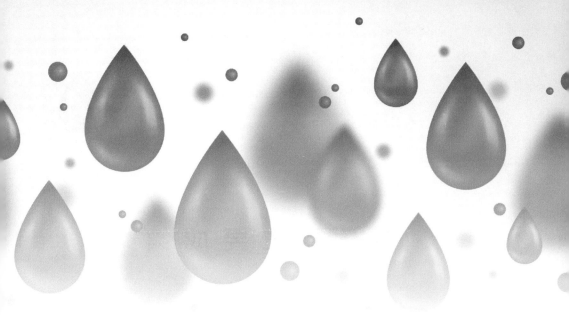

第八篇

———————————

总结与展望

———————————

第一章 主 要 成 绩

　　无偿献血是关系人民群众身体健康和生命安全的社会公益事业,党和政府历来高度重视。自1998年《中华人民共和国献血法》实施以来,在各级党委、政府和相关部门的组织领导和有力推动下,广大群众积极参与,我国全面建立无偿献血制度,血液管理法制体系和血站采供血服务体系日益完善。2019年我国无偿献血总人次达到1 562.3万人次,献血率达到11.2/千人口。2019年无偿献血总人次较去年增长4.0%。我国无偿献血工作体系基本完善,管理科学、保障有力、使用合理的无偿献血工作格局基本形成,各项工作实现跨越式发展。

一、血液管理法制化建设长效机制基本形成

　　2019年,国家卫生健康委继续坚持"开源、节流、保安全"的工作思路,以"提升依法治理水平、提升血液供应水平、提升血液安全水平、提升合理用血水平"的"四提升"为主线。不断健全法律体系,围绕《中华人民共和国献血法》《血站管理办法》《医疗机构临床用血管理办法》等,不断更新相关法规规范和技术标准。不断健全血液质量控制体系,完善血站、单采血浆站技术规程、标准和规范,加强人员培训和考核,提高专业人才队伍素质,指导血站、单采血浆站建立覆盖采供血全过程的血液管理质量控制与持续改进体系,定期开展内审和实验室室间质量评价,血液质量管理水平持续提升,血液报废率、血液质量相关不良事件持续下降并保持较低水平。

二、血液信息化管理和服务水平有效提高

强化血液安全信息化建设,提高信息化服务水平。2019 年我国血液管理信息系统及省级血液管理信息系统基本建成,实现血站全覆盖。长三角血液信息一体化建设、京津冀血液信息联网等部分区域建成区域性信息化管理平台,建立献血者档案共享数据库,实现用血异地减免、血液调剂、不合格献血者屏蔽、稀有血型献血者资源共享等。部分省份建成省级用血减免平台,形成"以医疗机构减免为主、网络减免为辅"的无偿献血者及亲属用血费用"一站式"减免的模式。依托信息化管理强化服务能力,提高服务水平。

三、采供血服务能力持续加强

我国已建成以血液中心、中心血站为主体,边远地区县级中心血库为补充,覆盖城乡、运行高效的血站服务体系。2019 年进一步强化血液预警和调配机制,基本解决季节性、区域性、偏型性血液供应紧张的世界难题。

健全血站技术规程、标准和规范,推进信息化建设,完善血站采供血全程质量管理体系,建立高危献血人员屏蔽制度和血液运输存储冷链管理制度,定期开展血站内审和实验室室间质量评价,血液报废率、血液质量相关不良事件持续下降并保持在较低水平。全面落实血液核酸检测策略,有效缩短人类免疫缺陷病毒(HIV)、乙型肝炎病毒、丙型肝炎病毒检测的"窗口期",基本阻断HIV 等重点传染病经输血途径传播。

2019 年底,基本实现原料血浆核酸检测全覆盖。彰显我国血液安全保障能力迈上新台阶。

四、血液安全技术保障能力持续提高

各地成立临床用血质量控制中心,健全临床用血培训、监督、管理、评价和通报制度,将临床用血作为医疗质量评价的重要指标。推广合理用血理念和经验,规范用血标准,严格用血指征,引导医疗机构加强患者血液管理,普及科学合理输血策略,推广自体血回输等血液保护技术,减少术中出血和异体输血不良反应的发生。近 5 年来,出院患者人均用血量、手术台均用血量分别降低20% 和 30%、自体血回输比例增长 30%。

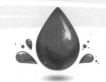

第二章　面　临　挑　战

　　血液供应和血液安全是开展临床医疗、维护人民群众健康的重要基础。《中华人民共和国献血法》实施二十余年来,我国血液安全管理水平快速提高,但传统和新增血液安全风险依然存在,伴随着全面推进小康社会的建设和"健康中国"建设的不断深化,社会对血液安全保障能力要求的不断提高,血液安全仍面临挑战。

一、血站资源布局结构有待优化

　　基层血站投入不足,服务能力和服务水平有待提高,中西部地区尤为突出,中小血站建设及服务质量不高,不同层次的血站功能定位有进一步优化的空间,基层采供血机构的血液安全保障能力面临挑战。

二、血站从业人员激励机制有待完善

　　血站从业人员激励保障措施急需提高,部分血站人员流失问题已影响到采供血工作的正常进行。采供血机构普遍缺乏科学合理的绩效结构,有些地区出现工作量与职工绩效脱节甚至背离的情况,不能在经济激励方面给予充分的保障。采供血一线业务人员、高层次专业技术人员绩效待遇与其他职工差距不大,造成急难险重和技术含量高的岗位工作积极性不高。专业技术人员受编制和岗位设置数量的限制,高职低聘现象普遍存在,在一定程度上影响和制约了采供血从业人员的工作积极性和能动性。

三、血液安全学科建设不足,专业人才缺乏

与发达国家相比,我国输血医学的学科建设相对滞后,目前,还没有输血医学或血液安全相关专业的高等教育人才培养体系,血液从业人员大多数为临床其他专业改行,也没有专业的继续教育保障体系。输血医学是一门多学科的医学交叉学科,同发达国家相比,我国输血医学起步并不晚,但发展缓慢,与发达国家的差距依然较大,与目前我国社会经济的发展不平衡,与临床医学各学科的发展也不匹配,在一定程度上影响到临床血液供应及输血安全。

四、血液安全风险预警能力有待加强

血液预警是通过监测输(献)血相关不良事件的发生,分析原因并提出处理和预防措施,不断提高输血技术和血液安全管理水平。自 20 世纪法国输血案发生以来,在美、英等发达国家广泛采用,是世界卫生组织推荐的最有效、最经济的血液安全科学保障措施。目前我国尚没有建立覆盖全国的血液安全风险预警体系,血液安全风险的早期干预和提前预警机制需要加强。我国现行法律法规尚缺乏对建立血液预警系统的明确支撑,尚未形成以数据为基础的血液安全风险发生、原因分析及政策建议的分析报告,为政府部门制定输血和血液安全相关政策的科学依据有待进一步加强。

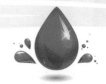

第三章　展　　望

一、进一步加强无偿献血宣传动员

无偿献血是一项社会性很强的医疗卫生事业,各级地方政府需要进一步健全"政府领导、部门合作、全社会参与"的无偿献血长效工作机制,营造无偿献血的良好社会氛围,充分发挥红十字会等社会团体体系优势,做好党政机关、企事业单位、高校、社区等无偿献血组织动员工作,不断扩大无偿献血者和志愿服务者队伍,进一步强化个人自愿无偿献血和团体自愿无偿献血协同发展的献血模式,提高血液供应保障能力。

二、强化血液管理信息网络建设

全面加强血液管理信息化建设,实现从献血者血管到用血者血管全链条的血液信息化管理。逐步推进血站、浆站、医疗机构及疾病控制等相关部门的联网运作,信息互通,有效屏蔽高危献血人群,普及电子无偿献血证,全面推广网上办理临床用血减免工作等,实现血液全流程信息化管理。提升血液供应保障服务能力。

三、提升血液安全风险管理能力

加强血液安全风险管理,推进输(献)血不良反应监测,建立血液安全风险研判、评估、决策和防控机制。进一步强化采供血机构全面质量管理建设,提升采供血机构血液质量管理能力;推进血液筛查技术和策略研究,提高经血传播病原体检测能力储备;开展血液联动保障机制建设,进一步提高血液供需平衡能力;精准开展医疗机构临床合理用血评价,提升临床用血风险控制能力。

四、创新血液安全人才培养模式

推动血液安全专业人才培养,设置合理的专业课程体系,明确培养方向,培养不同层次复合型血液安全专业人才。加强血液安全相关知识和法规培训,提升专业人员技能。加大血站从业人员在岗培训,持续开展岗前培训和在职继续教育。

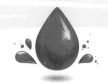

附　录

附表1　2019年千人口献血率汇总表

序号	地区	千人口献血率 / （千人口 $^{-1}$）	比2018年增长	
			增长情况 / （千人口 $^{-1}$）	增长率 / %
1	北京	18.7	2.4	14.9
2	天津	12.7	0.5	4.4
3	河北	11.2	0.6	5.6
4	山西	10.6	0.7	7.5
5	内蒙古	8.6	−0.1	−0.9
6	辽宁	9.7	−0.1	−1.2
7	吉林	10.5	0.6	6.5
8	黑龙江	10.8	0.8	8.5
9	上海	14.9	0.0	0.1
10	江苏	13.7	0.7	5.7
11	浙江	13.1	0.7	5.5
12	安徽	8.3	0.5	6.0
13	福建	9.1	0.4	4.3
14	江西	9.1	0.5	6.3
15	山东	10.8	0.5	4.5

续表

序号	地区	千人口献血率 / （千人口 -1）	比 2018 年增长	
			增长情况 / （千人口 -1）	增长率 / %
16	河南	12.7	0.4	3.3
17	湖北	11.9	0.2	2.1
18	湖南	9.0	0.4	4.4
19	广东	12.7	0.7	5.6
20	广西	11.9	0.7	6.5
21	海南	12.3	1.0	8.7
22	重庆	11.5	0.5	4.3
23	四川	10.0	0.8	8.5
24	贵州	10.8	0.6	5.4
25	云南	11.0	0.8	8.2
26	西藏	1.3	0.9	188.5
27	陕西	13.0	0.7	5.6
28	甘肃	8.2	0.1	1.1
29	青海	8.0	0.3	4.6
30	宁夏	9.8	0.4	4.0
31	新疆	6.8	0.5	7.3
32	兵团	5.3	-0.6	-9.9

附表 2　2019 年血液采集量情况汇总表

序号	地区	全血			血小板		
		全血 / 万 U	比 2018 年增长		血小板 / 万治疗量	比 2018 年增长	
			增长情况 / 万 U	增长率 / %		增长情况 / 万治疗量	增长率 / %
1	北京	55.9	5.3	10.5	11.2	2.4	26.8
2	天津	37.2	8.3	28.8	6.0	0.5	9.0
3	河北	144.4	7.9	5.8	12.2	1.4	12.7
4	山西	70.0	4.6	7.0	5.1	1.1	26.9
5	内蒙古	35.9	-0.4	-1.2	2.2	0.1	7.1

续表

序号	地区	全血			血小板		
		全血/万U	比2018年增长		血小板/万治疗量	比2018年增长	
			增长情况/万U	增长率/%		增长情况/万治疗量	增长率/%
6	辽宁	68.8	−1.8	−2.6	5.2	−0.1	−1.5
7	吉林	45.6	3.2	7.4	3.0	0.2	8.2
8	黑龙江	68.8	5.1	8.0	3.6	−0.1	−1.6
9	上海	46.3	0.6	1.3	4.9	0.3	7.6
10	江苏	163.6	10.8	7.1	18.6	2.2	13.1
11	浙江	107.7	7.4	7.4	14.2	4.6	47.4
12	安徽	80.8	4.4	5.8	4.3	0.5	14.6
13	福建	55.2	2.3	4.3	3.9	0.2	5.3
14	江西	68.0	4.2	6.6	5.1	0.8	19.0
15	山东	175.1	8.4	5.0	14.1	1.3	10.2
16	河南	217.8	7.1	3.4	17.3	1.5	9.3
17	湖北	105.1	1.4	1.4	11.9	1.5	14.7
18	湖南	103.3	5.3	5.5	7.7	0.9	13.9
19	广东	210.4	12.4	6.3	19.3	3.5	22.4
20	广西	94.5	5.6	6.3	5.4	0.7	14.9
21	海南	17.6	1.4	8.9	1.3	0.2	14.9
22	重庆	53.8	1.9	3.7	3.0	0.1	3.6
23	四川	133.8	9.8	7.9	6.0	1.0	19.4
24	贵州	59.1	2.7	4.9	3.2	0.5	17.5
25	云南	79.3	6.9	9.5	4.5	0.9	26.3
26	西藏	0.5	0.4	210.6	0.0	0.0	—
27	陕西	81.4	4.8	6.3	5.0	0.7	16.5
28	甘肃	31.5	0.6	2.0	1.6	0.2	15.1
29	青海	8.4	0.3	3.7	2.2	−0.5	−17.6
30	宁夏	12.2	0.5	4.7	0.6	0.1	10.8
31	新疆	26.2	1.8	7.3	2.9	0.8	37.8
32	兵团	2.6	−0.2	−7.2	0.1	0.0	33.3

附表 3　2019 年个人献血比例情况汇总表

序号	地区	比例 /%	比 2018 年增长	
			增长情况 / 百分点	增长率 /%
1	北京	70.3	0.0	−0.1
2	天津	81.9	−3.2	−3.7
3	河北	81.0	2.6	3.3
4	山西	78.6	−1.7	−2.1
5	内蒙古	83.5	−1.7	−2.0
6	辽宁	73.8	−3.3	−4.3
7	吉林	70.3	−0.3	−0.5
8	黑龙江	82.0	−1.0	−1.2
9	上海	36.6	1.0	2.9
10	江苏	65.1	1.0	1.6
11	浙江	50.2	−1.6	−3.1
12	安徽	81.9	3.2	4.1
13	福建	56.1	−4.4	−7.3
14	江西	65.8	−0.1	−0.2
15	山东	80.1	−0.5	−0.6
16	河南	71.9	−11.2	−13.5
17	湖北	87.4	−0.2	−0.2
18	湖南	72.5	0.7	1.0
19	广东	62.4	3.2	5.5
20	广西	72.5	−2.0	−2.7
21	海南	71.8	8.3	13.0
22	重庆	83.9	−0.5	−0.5
23	四川	56.9	−5.9	−9.4
24	贵州	83.2	−0.3	−0.4
25	云南	62.8	−1.9	−2.9
26	西藏	64.3	19.9	44.7
27	陕西	82.9	−1.4	−1.7
28	甘肃	74.7	4.1	5.8
29	青海	83.3	−0.6	−0.8
30	宁夏	76.3	−7.4	−8.9
31	新疆	87.2	2.7	3.2
32	兵团	99.2	0.0	0.0

附表 4　2019 年献血 400ml 占比情况汇总表

序号	地区	占比 /%	比 2018 年增长	
			增长情况 / 百分点	增长率 /%
1	北京	64.9	-2.9	-4.3
2	天津	76.2	-2.7	-3.5
3	河北	80.6	-0.3	-0.4
4	山西	90.3	0.4	0.4
5	内蒙古	66.7	-0.4	-0.7
6	辽宁	73.3	-1.6	-2.2
7	吉林	55.9	0.4	0.7
8	黑龙江	76.2	-4.7	-5.9
9	上海	38.5	1.7	4.6
10	江苏	41.7	3.1	8.0
11	浙江	37.5	-0.4	-1.1
12	安徽	49.0	-1.7	-3.3
13	福建	45.7	-3.3	-6.7
14	江西	56.7	-1.1	-2.0
15	山东	62.6	-0.4	-0.7
16	河南	91.1	-1.5	-1.6
17	湖北	47.2	-2.6	-5.2
18	湖南	57.9	3.9	7.2
19	广东	45.0	-0.2	-0.3
20	广西	57.0	-2.5	-4.2
21	海南	42.9	-9.3	-17.8
22	重庆	52.4	-2.1	-3.9
23	四川	46.6	-3.9	-7.7
24	贵州	55.1	-1.2	-2.1
25	云南	36.9	2.2	6.4
26	西藏	1.6	-3.6	-68.7
27	陕西	67.2	-0.1	-0.2
28	甘肃	29.1	-4.2	-12.6
29	青海	79.7	-1.3	-1.7
30	宁夏	82.7	-0.4	-0.4
31	新疆	39.8	-15.1	-27.5
32	兵团	34.8	-2.9	-7.6

附表 5 2019 年保密性弃血占比情况汇总表

序号	地区	保密性弃血 /(人次·万⁻¹)	比 2018 年增长	
			增长情况 /(人次 / 万⁻¹)	增长 /%
1	北京	1.01	0.13	14.74
2	天津	0.45	−0.22	−33.23
3	河北	0.18	−0.05	−22.51
4	山西	11.06	10.03	973.69
5	内蒙古	5.19	5.14	9 873.90
6	辽宁	0.16	−4.98	−96.98
7	吉林	0.23	0.19	518.37
8	黑龙江	0.12	−0.40	−76.41
9	上海	0.57	0.11	23.76
10	江苏	0.69	0.28	67.83
11	浙江	0.66	0.34	105.25
12	安徽	0.47	−13.07	−96.56
13	福建	1.23	0.64	108.76
14	江西	0.28	0.17	167.33
15	山东	0.04	−0.31	−87.20
16	河南	0.08	0.00	−3.65
17	湖北	0.55	−0.13	−18.65
18	湖南	0.17	−0.11	−39.82
19	广东	2.26	−0.29	−11.30
20	广西	0.23	−21.63	−98.97
21	海南	0.00	0.00	—
22	重庆	7.28	6.80	1 432.25
23	四川	0.80	0.31	63.34
24	贵州	0.46	−0.38	−45.12
25	云南	0.74	0.47	179.98
26	西藏	20.62	−2.84	−12.09
27	陕西	0.07	0.02	40.38
28	甘肃	24.99	12.86	105.98
29	青海	9.41	4.84	105.88
30	宁夏	0.24	−3.18	−93.11
31	新疆	0.00	−0.17	−100.00
32	兵团	0.55	0.03	6.35

附表 6 2019 年女性献血者比例情况汇总表

序号	地区	比例 /%	比 2018 年增长	
			增长情况 / 百分点	增长率 /%
1	北京	31.3	0.6	2.0
2	天津	26.2	0.6	2.2
3	河北	33.8	0.4	1.3
4	山西	29.8	−0.4	−1.2
5	内蒙古	34.9	0.1	0.3
6	辽宁	39.5	−0.1	−0.2
7	吉林	37.5	0.8	2.2
8	黑龙江	41.0	0.5	1.3
9	上海	32.2	1.8	5.8
10	江苏	40.1	0.6	1.6
11	浙江	39.0	0.7	1.9
12	安徽	40.5	0.2	0.4
13	福建	38.1	0.3	0.8
14	江西	39.5	0.5	1.3
15	山东	30.1	0.4	1.4
16	河南	37.0	0.0	−0.1
17	湖北	38.7	0.6	1.6
18	湖南	39.8	0.2	0.6
19	广东	32.2	0.6	2.0
20	广西	35.3	0.5	1.4
21	海南	29.8	−1.0	−3.4
22	重庆	50.1	−0.5	−1.0
23	四川	48.7	0.6	1.2
24	贵州	51.8	0.4	0.8
25	云南	45.3	0.6	1.4
26	西藏	26.8	1.1	4.3
27	陕西	37.8	0.2	0.4
28	甘肃	32.4	1.3	4.2
29	青海	32.8	−0.9	−2.8
30	宁夏	36.8	0.3	0.8
31	新疆	33.9	0.0	0.1
32	兵团	35.6	0.9	2.7

附表 7　2019 年 18~35 岁献血者占比情况汇总表

序号	地区	占比 /%	比 2018 年增长	
			增长情况 / 百分点	增长率 /%
1	北京	64.3	−0.6	−0.9
2	天津	70.6	0.1	0.1
3	河北	45.7	−0.4	−1.0
4	山西	43.8	0.8	1.9
5	内蒙古	45.5	−0.3	−0.6
6	辽宁	48.8	0.8	1.6
7	吉林	51.9	1.6	3.2
8	黑龙江	42.2	1.2	3.1
9	上海	72.8	−0.6	−0.8
10	江苏	50.5	−0.4	−0.8
11	浙江	53.3	−0.4	−0.7
12	安徽	52.0	0.0	0.0
13	福建	52.5	0.3	0.5
14	江西	56.1	0.0	0.1
15	山东	52.3	−0.3	−0.6
16	河南	40.6	0.5	1.2
17	湖北	51.5	−1.4	−2.6
18	湖南	55.2	0.6	1.2
19	广东	63.1	−0.5	−0.8
20	广西	55.4	1.7	3.2
21	海南	60.7	−2.4	−3.8
22	重庆	49.2	−0.4	−0.8
23	四川	43.1	0.0	0.1
24	贵州	56.5	0.3	0.6
25	云南	61.4	0.7	1.2
26	西藏	78.1	9.3	13.6
27	陕西	53.8	−0.2	−0.4
28	甘肃	57.9	−0.2	−0.3
29	青海	47.0	1.0	2.1
30	宁夏	57.1	1.8	3.3
31	新疆	59.9	2.6	4.5
32	兵团	56.7	−0.2	−0.4

附表 8　2019 年本科以上学历献血者占比情况汇总表

序号	地区	占比 /%	比 2018 年增长	
			增长情况 / 百分点	增长率 /%
1	北京	38.4	3.8	10.8
2	天津	25.9	2.9	12.4
3	河北	15.2	−0.1	−0.4
4	山西	21.3	2.1	11.0
5	内蒙古	23.6	0.4	1.6
6	辽宁	24.5	3.5	16.7
7	吉林	27.8	3.6	14.9
8	黑龙江	22.3	1.1	5.1
9	上海	26.2	2.8	11.9
10	江苏	22.0	0.5	2.2
11	浙江	20.3	−1.9	−8.7
12	安徽	26.0	1.4	5.7
13	福建	32.3	3.1	10.7
14	江西	26.1	0.6	2.3
15	山东	20.8	1.0	4.9
16	河南	15.1	1.4	10.1
17	湖北	26.2	−0.8	−3.1
18	湖南	28.7	−0.1	−0.5
19	广东	18.7	−0.6	−3.0
20	广西	20.0	1.7	9.3
21	海南	27.6	−1.1	−3.9
22	重庆	21.0	0.0	−0.1
23	四川	17.9	0.7	4.2
24	贵州	15.7	−0.2	−1.3
25	云南	26.0	1.8	7.2
26	西藏	32.9	11.5	53.9
27	陕西	22.6	1.0	4.6
28	甘肃	20.9	1.5	7.6
29	青海	20.1	0.5	2.6
30	宁夏	23.8	3.7	18.5
31	新疆	22.4	2.6	12.9
32	兵团	26.4	0.1	0.3

附表 9　2019 年血站血液检测情况汇总表

序号	地区	检测总数			不合格数			不合格率	
		检测总数 /万人次	比 2018 年增长		不合格数 /万人次	比 2018 年增长		不合格率 /%	比 2018 年增长
			增长数 /万人次	增长比例 /%		增长数 /万人次	增长比例 /%		增长情况 /百分点
1	北京	47.5	6.3	15.3	7.4	1.3	21.3	15.5	0.8
2	天津	22.8	1.0	4.6	2.9	0.2	6.2	12.8	0.2
3	河北	94.6	4.9	5.4	11.5	1.1	10.8	12.1	0.6
4	山西	44.7	2.7	6.4	6.0	−0.2	−2.8	13.5	−1.3
5	内蒙古	22.8	0.6	2.5	2.6	0.1	6.2	11.2	0.4
6	辽宁	47.8	−11.0	−18.7	7.8	−0.1	−1.8	16.4	2.8
7	吉林	31.4	1.6	5.4	3.3	0.1	4.5	10.5	−0.1
8	黑龙江	41.9	0.5	1.2	3.8	−0.6	−12.9	9.1	−1.5
9	上海	35.7	7.8	27.8	3.9	−0.3	−6.4	10.8	−4.0
10	江苏	119.8	8.1	7.2	9.4	−0.1	−0.7	7.8	−0.6
11	浙江	86.1	5.0	6.1	12.3	1.6	15.0	14.2	1.1
12	安徽	55.7	3.1	6.0	4.3	0.1	1.3	7.8	−0.4
13	福建	39.8	1.2	3.2	4.5	−1.1	−20.0	11.3	−3.3
14	江西	44.2	1.3	3.0	3.4	−0.4	−10.0	7.8	−1.1
15	山东	116.5	5.5	4.9	10.5	0.9	9.0	9.0	0.3
16	河南	131.3	3.6	2.8	14.4	1.8	14.0	11.0	1.1
17	湖北	69.1	−0.8	−1.2	4.3	0.2	4.2	6.3	0.3
18	湖南	64.7	2.8	4.6	3.9	−0.4	−8.2	6.1	−0.9
19	广东	158.6	11.4	7.8	19.6	1.4	7.6	12.3	0.0
20	广西	64.2	3.1	5.0	6.9	0.7	11.2	10.8	0.6
21	海南	13.2	1.1	8.8	1.9	0.0	0.0	14.2	−1.2
22	重庆	40.9	2.1	5.3	5.6	0.0	−0.7	13.6	−0.8
23	四川	85.7	0.5	0.6	10.5	0.0	−0.2	12.2	−0.1

序号	地区	检测总数			不合格数			不合格率	
		检测总数/万人次	比 2018 年增长		不合格数/万人次	比 2018 年增长		不合格率/%	比 2018 年增长
			增长数/万人次	增长比例/%		增长数/万人次	增长比例/%		增长情况/百分点
24	贵州	41.9	2.4	6.0	4.4	0.6	14.9	10.5	0.8
25	云南	56.5	1.7	3.1	6.5	−0.5	−7.7	11.5	−1.4
26	西藏	0.5	0.2	77.4	0.1	0.0	−22.8	21.8	−28.3
27	陕西	53.4	2.3	4.6	3.9	−0.4	−9.6	7.3	−1.2
28	甘肃	26.9	4.4	19.3	1.9	−0.4	−18.4	6.9	−3.2
29	青海	5.9	0.2	3.2	1.3	0.0	2.3	21.4	−0.2
30	宁夏	7.9	0.5	7.1	1.4	0.3	23.0	17.8	2.3
31	新疆	18.4	0.8	4.5	2.4	0.2	9.7	13.2	0.6
32	兵团	1.7	−0.3	−15.5	0.2	−0.1	−30.3	10.6	−2.2

附表 10　2019 年献血前血液检测情况汇总表

序号	地区	检测总数			不合格数			不合格率	
		检测总数/万人次	比 2018 年增长		不合格数/万人次	比 2018 年增长		不合格率/%	比 2018 年增长
			增长数/万人次	增长比例/%		增长数/万人次	增长比例/%		增长情况/百分点
1	北京	47.5	6.3	15.3	6.6	1.2	22.2	13.9	0.8
2	天津	22.8	1.0	4.6	2.6	0.1	5.0	11.6	0.0
3	河北	94.6	4.9	5.4	10.3	1.0	11.0	10.9	0.5
4	山西	44.7	2.7	6.4	5.1	−0.2	−4.2	11.4	−1.3
5	内蒙古	22.8	0.6	2.5	2.0	0.1	5.1	8.7	0.2
6	辽宁	47.8	−11.0	−18.7	7.3	−0.1	−1.0	15.2	2.7
7	吉林	31.4	1.6	5.4	2.9	0.1	4.3	9.1	−0.1
8	黑龙江	41.9	0.5	1.2	3.1	−0.6	−16.8	7.5	−1.6
9	上海	35.7	7.8	27.8	2.3	−0.5	−17.4	6.5	−3.6

续表

序号	地区	检测总数			不合格数			不合格率	
		检测总数 / 万人次	比2018年增长		不合格数 / 万人次	比2018年增长		不合格率 / %	比2018年增长
			增长数 / 万人次	增长比例 / %		增长数 / 万人次	增长比例 / %		增长情况 / 百分点
10	江苏	119.8	8.1	7.2	8.0	−0.1	−1.1	6.7	−0.6
11	浙江	86.1	5.0	6.1	11.2	1.6	16.1	13.0	1.1
12	安徽	55.7	3.1	6.0	3.1	−0.1	−3.5	5.6	−0.6
13	福建	39.8	1.2	3.2	3.7	−1.1	−23.2	9.4	−3.2
14	江西	44.2	1.3	3.0	2.7	−0.4	−12.7	6.0	−1.1
15	山东	116.5	5.5	4.9	8.8	1.0	12.5	7.6	0.5
16	河南	131.3	3.6	2.8	11.6	0.9	8.1	8.9	0.4
17	湖北	69.1	−0.8	−1.2	2.8	0.1	3.0	4.0	0.2
18	湖南	64.7	2.8	4.6	2.6	−0.3	−9.7	4.1	−0.6
19	广东	158.6	11.4	7.8	14.8	0.7	5.1	9.3	−0.2
20	广西	64.2	3.1	5.0	5.5	0.6	12.3	8.6	0.6
21	海南	13.2	1.1	8.8	1.6	0.0	1.9	12.2	−0.8
22	重庆	40.9	2.1	5.3	4.7	0.0	−0.3	11.4	−0.6
23	四川	85.7	0.5	0.6	7.2	−0.4	−5.8	8.4	−0.6
24	贵州	41.9	2.4	6.0	3.2	0.5	17.0	7.6	0.7
25	云南	56.5	1.7	3.1	5.3	−0.6	−10.1	9.4	−1.4
26	西藏	0.5	0.2	77.4	0.1	0.0	−25.5	20.1	−27.7
27	陕西	53.4	2.3	4.6	2.9	−0.5	−15.0	5.5	−1.3
28	甘肃	26.9	4.4	19.3	1.4	−0.4	−23.9	5.3	−3.0
29	青海	5.9	0.2	3.2	1.1	0.0	−0.3	18.9	−0.7
30	宁夏	7.9	0.5	7.1	1.3	0.3	23.7	16.8	2.3
31	新疆	18.4	0.8	4.5	2.0	0.2	10.9	11.1	0.6
32	兵团	1.7	−0.3	−15.5	0.1	−0.1	−37.2	7.4	−2.5

附表 11　2019 年血液实验室检测情况汇总表

序号	地区	检测总数			不合格数			不合格率	
		检测总数 / 万份	比 2018 年增长		不合格数 / 万份	比 2018 年增长		不合格率 /%	比 2018 年增长
			增长数 / 万份	增长情况 /%		增长数 / 万份	增长情况 /%		增长情况 / 百分点
1	北京	41.9	5.4	14.8	0.8	0.1	14.3	1.9	0.0
2	天津	19.8	0.9	4.8	0.3	0.0	19.8	1.4	0.2
3	河北	85.3	5.4	6.7	1.1	0.1	9.3	1.3	0.0
4	山西	40.6	2.8	7.5	0.9	0.1	6.2	2.2	0.0
5	内蒙古	22.9	0.0	−0.2	0.6	0.1	10.3	2.5	0.2
6	辽宁	43.0	0.3	0.8	0.6	−0.1	−10.3	1.3	−0.2
7	吉林	29.0	2.2	8.0	0.4	0.0	6.3	1.5	0.0
8	黑龙江	41.0	3.0	8.0	0.7	0.1	12.4	1.6	0.1
9	上海	35.1	0.3	0.8	1.5	0.2	17.0	4.4	0.6
10	江苏	114.8	10.1	9.7	1.4	0.0	1.8	1.2	−0.1
11	浙江	75.9	4.8	6.8	1.0	0.0	4.3	1.4	0.0
12	安徽	52.9	3.2	6.4	1.2	0.2	16.3	2.3	0.2
13	福建	35.9	1.6	4.5	0.8	0.0	−0.7	2.2	−0.1
14	江西	41.8	2.2	5.6	0.8	0.0	1.0	1.9	−0.1
15	山东	109.4	5.4	5.2	1.7	−0.1	−6.2	1.6	−0.2
16	河南	178.0	56.9	46.9	2.8	0.9	47.5	1.6	0.0
17	湖北	71.1	−0.8	−1.1	1.5	0.1	6.5	2.1	0.2
18	湖南	62.2	2.6	4.4	1.3	−0.1	−5.2	2.1	−0.2
19	广东	153.6	12.6	8.9	4.8	0.7	16.0	3.1	0.2
20	广西	63.2	3.1	5.1	1.4	0.1	7.0	2.2	0.0
21	海南	11.5	0.9	8.7	0.3	0.0	−10.1	2.3	−0.5
22	重庆	36.3	2.1	6.0	0.9	0.0	−2.9	2.5	−0.2

续表

序号	地区	检测总数			不合格数			不合格率	
		检测总数/万份	比2018年增长		不合格数/万份	比2018年增长		不合格率/%	比2018年增长
			增长数/万份	增长情况/%		增长数/万份	增长情况/%		增长情况/百分点
23	四川	83.9	7.0	9.1	3.3	0.4	14.9	3.9	0.2
24	贵州	42.3	2.6	6.4	1.2	0.1	9.7	2.9	0.1
25	云南	52.9	4.3	8.9	1.2	0.1	5.2	2.2	−0.1
26	西藏	0.5	0.3	203.9	0.0	0.0	30.9	2.0	−2.6
27	陕西	50.3	2.8	5.9	1.0	0.1	11.7	1.9	0.1
28	甘肃	21.6	0.3	1.4	0.4	0.0	7.0	2.0	0.1
29	青海	5.0	0.2	4.6	0.1	0.0	27.6	2.9	0.5
30	宁夏	6.8	0.3	5.2	0.1	0.0	13.0	1.1	0.1
31	新疆	17.3	−0.7	−3.8	0.4	0.0	3.6	2.2	0.2
32	兵团	1.5	−0.2	−13.7	0.1	0.0	−6.9	3.5	0.3

附表12　2019年血液成分分离比例情况汇总表

序号	地区	分离比例/%	比2018年增长	
			增长情况/百分点	增长率/%
1	北京	100.00	0.00	0.00
2	天津	99.96	0.14	0.14
3	河北	99.83	0.13	0.13
4	山西	99.26	−0.46	−0.46
5	内蒙古	99.81	0.49	0.49
6	辽宁	99.87	0.01	0.01
7	吉林	99.89	0.02	0.02
8	黑龙江	99.44	0.41	0.41
9	上海	99.88	0.02	0.02

续表

序号	地区	分离比例 /%	比 2018 年增长	
			增长情况 / 百分点	增长率 /%
10	江苏	99.98	0.01	0.01
11	浙江	99.92	0.04	0.04
12	安徽	99.91	0.05	0.05
13	福建	100.00	0.03	0.03
14	江西	100.00	0.00	0.00
15	山东	99.94	0.04	0.04
16	河南	99.83	0.01	0.01
17	湖北	99.95	0.01	0.01
18	湖南	100.00	0.00	0.00
19	广东	99.86	−0.12	−0.12
20	广西	99.84	−0.14	−0.14
21	海南	99.98	−0.02	−0.02
22	重庆	99.94	0.27	0.27
23	四川	99.98	0.00	0.00
24	贵州	99.96	0.01	0.01
25	云南	100.00	0.00	0.00
26	西藏	93.42	−4.44	−4.54
27	陕西	99.94	0.03	0.03
28	甘肃	99.85	0.09	0.09
29	青海	98.47	−1.13	−1.13
30	宁夏	99.97	2.75	2.82
31	新疆	99.62	2.81	2.91
32	兵团	99.63	1.94	1.98

附表 13　2019 年浓缩血小板分离率情况汇总表

序号	地区	分离率 /%	比 2018 年增长	
			增长情况 / 百分点	增长率 /%
1	北京	0.5	−5.7	−91.4
2	天津	12.1	1.5	13.8
3	河北	0.2	0.0	2.2
4	山西	0.6	−0.1	−16.5
5	内蒙古	6.4	−2.1	−24.3
6	辽宁	0.1	0.1	—
7	吉林	0.5	−0.4	−42.6
8	黑龙江	0.3	0.1	54.0
9	上海	1.5	0.6	61.1
10	江苏	0.3	0.1	57.5
11	浙江	0.2	−0.1	−31.2
12	安徽	4.3	−0.8	−15.1
13	福建	4.5	3.5	346.5
14	江西	1.7	1.1	205.1
15	山东	0.0	0.0	73.1
16	河南	0.5	0.3	134.7
17	湖北	0.0	−0.1	−100.0
18	湖南	9.8	0.7	7.2
19	广东	3.8	−3.9	−50.3
20	广西	2.6	0.0	−0.8
21	海南	0.0	0.0	—
22	重庆	0.2	0.1	232.4
23	四川	6.5	−0.6	−7.9
24	贵州	0.8	−0.2	−21.1
25	云南	0.0	0.0	−100.0
26	西藏	0.0	0.0	—
27	陕西	1.1	−0.1	−8.4
28	甘肃	0.0	0.0	−74.5
29	青海	3.1	−3.3	−51.6
30	宁夏	17.7	16.9	2 234.2
31	新疆	0.2	−0.3	−67.2
32	兵团	0.6	0.5	690.8

附表 14 2019 年供血总量情况汇总表

序号	地区	供血总量 / 万 U	比 2018 年增长	
			供血总量 / 万 U	增长率 /%
1	北京	138.5	10.4	8.2
2	天津	68.7	2.6	3.9
3	河北	275.4	24.3	9.7
4	山西	118.9	12.7	11.9
5	内蒙古	63.1	−2.6	−4.0
6	辽宁	135.1	8.0	6.3
7	吉林	92.5	13.7	17.4
8	黑龙江	125.7	3.0	2.5
9	上海	102.7	12.7	14.2
10	江苏	376.8	64.3	20.6
11	浙江	248.3	25.2	11.3
12	安徽	155.8	13.7	9.6
13	福建	121.0	23.9	24.6
14	江西	156.4	31.5	25.2
15	山东	352.7	40.9	13.1
16	河南	450.8	43.5	10.7
17	湖北	217.4	22.8	11.7
18	湖南	227.3	20.2	9.8
19	广东	487.0	41.1	9.2
20	广西	200.5	35.5	21.5
21	海南	36.7	8.8	31.6
22	重庆	111.5	11.7	11.7
23	四川	231.6	23.0	11.0
24	贵州	113.0	10.8	10.6
25	云南	161.3	25.6	18.9
26	西藏	2.9	1.9	194.4
27	陕西	166.2	20.1	13.7
28	甘肃	71.7	−65.9	−47.9
29	青海	19.5	0.9	4.7
30	宁夏	25.2	2.9	12.9
31	新疆	66.8	15.0	28.9
32	兵团	5.5	−2.9	−34.4

附表 15　2019 年人均用血量汇总表

序号	地区	人均用血量 /ml	比 2018 年增长	
			人均用血量 /ml	增长率 /%
1	北京	5.8	0.4	6.9
2	天津	3.7	0.1	2.6
3	河北	3.7	0.2	4.7
4	山西	3.7	0.3	8.3
5	内蒙古	2.9	0.1	2.6
6	辽宁	3.1	−0.1	−1.6
7	吉林	3.3	0.3	10.9
8	黑龙江	3.6	0.3	10.3
9	上海	3.6	0.1	3.7
10	江苏	4.2	0.5	12.8
11	浙江	3.6	0.2	5.6
12	安徽	2.5	0.1	5.5
13	福建	3.0	0.4	14.4
14	江西	2.9	0.2	7.9
15	山东	3.4	0.1	3.8
16	河南	4.5	0.2	3.8
17	湖北	3.5	0.1	2.4
18	湖南	2.9	0.2	6.4
19	广东	4.0	0.7	20.6
20	广西	3.8	0.3	9.8
21	海南	3.7	0.3	9.1
22	重庆	3.4	0.2	5.8
23	四川	3.0	0.2	8.0
24	贵州	3.2	0.1	4.0
25	云南	3.3	0.3	10.0
26	西藏	1.2	0.7	161.8
27	陕西	4.1	0.2	5.0
28	甘肃	2.5	0.2	8.0
29	青海	2.9	0.3	9.7
30	宁夏	3.5	0.1	2.9
31	新疆	2.1	0.1	6.6
32	兵团	1.8	0.0	−1.5

附表 16　2019 年万人血小板使用量汇总表

序号	地区	使用量 / 治疗量	比 2018 年增长	
			增长量 / 治疗量	增长率 /%
1	北京	63.115	10.904	20.9
2	天津	40.668	3.528	9.5
3	河北	15.849	1.576	11.0
4	山西	10.784	1.830	20.4
5	内蒙古	9.611	−0.970	−9.2
6	辽宁	11.718	−0.304	−2.5
7	吉林	11.121	0.900	8.8
8	黑龙江	9.790	0.066	0.7
9	上海	23.105	3.454	17.6
10	江苏	23.122	3.553	18.2
11	浙江	19.147	1.910	11.1
12	安徽	7.604	1.127	17.4
13	福建	11.085	1.564	16.4
14	江西	11.499	2.385	26.2
15	山东	14.000	1.271	10.0
16	河南	18.102	1.494	9.0
17	湖北	19.599	2.474	14.4
18	湖南	12.519	1.541	14.0
19	广东	18.251	3.079	20.3
20	广西	11.172	1.206	12.1
21	海南	13.742	1.731	14.4
22	重庆	9.474	0.418	4.6
23	四川	8.092	1.145	16.5
24	贵州	8.735	0.869	11.0

续表

序号	地区	使用量 / 治疗量	比 2018 年增长	
			增长量 / 治疗量	增长率 /%
25	云南	9.276	1.848	24.9
26	西藏	0.109	0.109	—
27	陕西	13.144	1.807	15.9
28	甘肃	5.734	0.659	13.0
29	青海	36.135	−8.508	−19.1
30	宁夏	11.305	3.543	45.6
31	新疆	9.237	1.944	26.7
32	兵团	3.529	0.552	18.6

附表 17 2019 年有形成分利用率情况汇总表

序号	地区	利用率 /%	比 2018 年增长	
			增长情况 / 百分点	增长率 /%
1	北京	100.5	−5.7	−5.4
2	天津	112.0	1.6	3.4
3	河北	100.0	0.1	0.3
4	山西	99.9	−0.6	−1.0
5	内蒙古	106.2	−1.6	−2.7
6	辽宁	100.0	0.1	0.3
7	吉林	100.4	−0.4	−0.7
8	黑龙江	99.7	0.5	1.0
9	上海	101.4	0.6	1.2
10	江苏	100.3	0.1	0.2
11	浙江	100.1	0.0	−0.1
12	安徽	104.2	−0.7	−1.3
13	福建	104.5	3.5	6.5

续表

序号	地区	利用率/%	比 2018 年增长	
			增长情况/百分点	增长率/%
14	江西	101.7	1.1	2.3
15	山东	100.0	0.1	0.1
16	河南	100.3	0.3	0.6
17	湖北	100.0	0.0	−0.1
18	湖南	109.8	0.7	1.3
19	广东	103.7	−4.0	−8.8
20	广西	102.4	−0.2	−0.3
21	海南	100.0	0.0	0.0
22	重庆	100.1	0.4	0.7
23	四川	106.5	−0.6	−0.9
24	贵州	100.7	−0.2	−0.3
25	云南	100.0	0.0	0.0
26	西藏	93.4	−4.4	−5.9
27	陕西	101.1	−0.1	−0.2
28	甘肃	99.9	0.1	0.3
29	青海	101.6	−4.5	−9.9
30	宁夏	117.7	19.7	38.9
31	新疆	99.8	2.5	5.5
32	兵团	100.2	2.4	7.6

China's Report on Blood Safety 2019

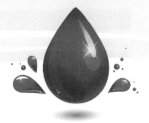

National Health Commission of the People's Republic of China

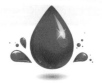

Introduction

The year 2019 was one of steady growth for China's national blood system. With the Healthy China Initiative in place, the Chinese government improved the safety, supply and quality of the blood services, providing more safeguard for the health of the people. Guided by the principles of optimizing blood management, improving quality control, strengthening safety surveillance and safeguarding patient health, a multi-pronged approach was adopted to enhance law-based governance, information management, publicity and institutional service capacity, pushing for further progress in China's national blood system.

To begin with, the number of voluntary non-remunerated blood donors and the volume of blood donation maintained a growing momentum. The blood donation rate reached 11.2 per 1,000 population in 2019, an increase of 0.1% over 2018. A total of 26.49 million units of blood were collected during the year, up by 5.7% from that of 2018.

On November 4, 2019, a *Notice on Promoting Non-remunerated Blood Donation* (hereinafter referred to as the *Notice*) was jointly issued by eleven ministries and departments of the Chinese central government, including the National Health Commission, the Publicity Department of the CPC Central Committee, the Central Commission for Guiding Cultural and Ethical Progress, the National Development and Reform Commission, the Ministry of Education, the Ministry of Finance, the Ministry of

Human Resources and Social Security, the Ministry of Housing and Urban-Rural Development, the National Federation of Trade Unions, the Red Cross Society of China and the Health Bureau of the Logistics and Support Department of the Central Military Commission. The Notice required sustained efforts for sound development of non-remunerated blood donation in China. The Notice also outlined the framework arrangements in establishing a multi-sectoral coordination mechanism, enhancing awareness and mobilization measures for non-remunerated blood donation, promoting standards for the blood collection and supply service and developing a long-term mechanism of donor incentives. It required health administrative departments at all levels to strengthen blood management in collaboration with the departments of finance, transportation, and urban development. The purpose was to guarantee better enforcement of the *Blood Donation Law of the People's Republic of China* and formulate a roadmap forward featuring government leadership, interdepartmental collaboration and public participation. These measures aimed at boosting the long-term mechanism of non-remunerated blood donation and contributing to the sustained development of blood collection and supply in China.

China's information network for blood management was improving rapidly in 2019. The National Blood Management Information System went on line officially, enabling accessibility of interconnected data and information among blood establishments across the country. Some provinces and municipalities established their own information systems for blood management, connecting and integrating all blood establishments within their jurisdictions. Meanwhile, inter-network connectivity between blood establishments and medical institutions were being realized in some cities. The integrated information management systems allowed the blood collection, preparation, storage, transportation and clinical use processes to operate in a safer and more controllable environment. Such provinces as Anhui, Guizhou, Hainan, Henan, Hunan, Jiangsu, Jiangxi, Shanghai, Tianjin, Zhejiang and Hebei gradually build their integrated platforms for blood cost reimbursement, reduction or exemption on top of the information systems. They formed a one-stop service model for non-remunerated blood donors and their relatives to get blood cost reimbursement, reduction or exemption primarily at medical institutions, but also through online schemes. Regional blood information networks such as those in the Yangtze River Delta and the Beijing-Tianjin-Hebei regions, which were gradually built and expanded, played an important role in keeping a blood donor registry, enabling long-distance reimbursement and exemption of blood expenses for donors, regulation of blood safety, screening of unqualified blood donors and donor resource sharing for rare blood types.

The capacities of blood collection and supply were reinforced. The number of people working in the national blood service reached 36,300, with the number of practitioners holding a bachelor's or above degree increasing further. The numbers rose by 1.62% and 0.24% respectively compared with those in 2018. Health technicians working at the blood establishments accounted for 73.43% of the total employees. The number of registered nurses increased by 1.17% over that of 2018. In 2019, the blood establishments cover a total area of 2.12 million square meters, with a total construction area of 2.05 million square meters. There were 45 more fixed blood collection sites, 8 more blood collection vehicles and 6 more blood delivery vehicles, increasing 3.09%, 0.51% and 0.40% over those of 2018.

Blood safety and availability were improved in the Three Regions and Three Prefectures (*see Section Seven*). With much attention and support from health departments at all levels, blood safety in these regions and prefectures witnessed much progress. Survey data from the five blood establishments in these regions and prefectures showed that the investments were on a steady rise. The total amount of transfer payments reached 24.205 million yuan in 2019, which was a 6-fold increase from that of 2015. Furthermore, the blood collection and supply capacities were also growing. In 2019, a total of 5,005 blood donations were collected at the blood establishments in these regions and prefectures, and the total volume of blood donation reached 8,038 units, an increase of 37.8% and 42.8% respectively over 2015. The utilization rate of blood components continued to rise, with erythrocyte and plasma reaching 10,312.3 and 7,411.5 units respectively, an increase of 29.5% and 35.6% compared with 2015.

Progress was made in managing the clinical use of blood. In 2019, the National Health Commission issued the *Quality Control Indicators for Clinical Use of Blood* (2019 Edition) (2019, No. 620) to regulate, from the national level, blood transfusion for clinical diagnosis and treatment. This measure aimed to promote standardized and rational use of blood in clinical settings and improve the service capacity and professionalism of blood transfusion departments. The National Health Commission adopted the national blood safety technical inspection as a starting point to strengthen the supervision of blood safety practices in all provinces. All provincial health departments conducted their own supervision and inspection of clinical use of blood at medical institutions under a unified framework of the National Health Commission. Provincial quality control centers relied on their increasing professional expertise to regulate the clinical use of blood by medical institutions within their jurisdictions.

(Remark: the data of this report do not include HONG KONG SAR, MACAO SAR and TAIWAN Province)

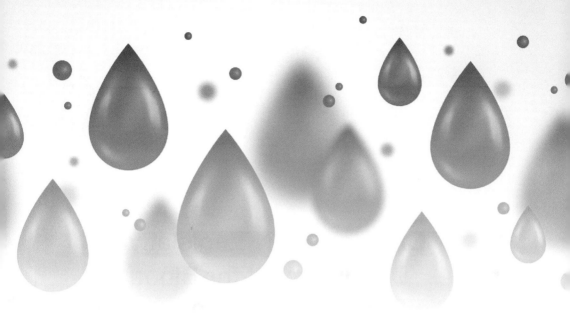

Section One

Blood Safety Management

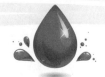

Chapter One   Legislative Development for Blood Management

I. Legal frameworks for blood management

Since the implementation of the *Blood Donation Law of the People's Republic of China* in 1998, the legislative development for blood management in China has grown rapidly. Legal frameworks and their contents have been constantly improved and updated centering on the system and capacity building of non-remunerated blood donation, blood collection and supply and clinical use of blood.

The implementation of the *Technical and Operational Procedures for Blood Establishments* (2015 Edition) has contributed significantly to the standardized management of blood establishments, realizing full coverage of nucleic acid testing and improving overall blood quality and safety. To better adapt to the growing technical requirements of blood establishments, the National Health Commission (NHC) issued the *Technical and Operational Procedures for Blood Establishments* (2019 Edition) on April 28, 2019. These new regulations made improvements with strengthened protection of the rights and interests of blood donors, enhancing blood collection technical standards, refining blood component preparation requirements, making adjustment to blood testing, and improving blood storage, distribution and transportation management and quality control. Higher standards and improvements over the previous framework enhanced the capacity of the blood establishments and contributed significantly to the development of the national blood system.

China's legal framework for blood management saw steady progress, forming a legal system with the *Blood Donation Law of the People's Republic of China* as the top policy, and other laws and regulations such as *Regulations on the Management of Blood Products*, *Measures for the Management of Blood Establishments*, and *Measures for the Management of Clinical Use of Blood at Medical Institutions* as the main pillars (Table 1-1).

II. Progress in raising blood technical standards

As the guiding documents on the blood collection and supply technology, blood standards play an irreplaceable role in improving the collection, supply and quality of blood at blood establishments, and transfusion and safety of blood for clinical use at medical institutions. In 2001, China's Standardization Administration and the former Ministry of Health approved and released three standards in this regard, i.e., GB 18467 *Health Examination Requirements for Blood Donors*, GB 18469 *Quality Requirements for Whole Blood and Constituent Blood*, and WS/T 203 *Commonly Used Terms for Blood Transfusion Medicine*. By 2019, a total of 12 standards were in place (Table 1-2). China is committed to building a solid system of blood standards, striving to make these standards forward-looking and constructive. By improving the blood standards system, a more powerful warrant for blood safety and patient health was gained.

The Technical Committee of Blood Standards under the State Health Standards Committee, led and supported by the NHC Department of Medical Affairs and Administration, Department of Laws and Regulations and the NHC Guidance Center for Medical Management Services, implemented the various tasks in an orderly manner, actively promoted the pilot project of blood group standards for advances in blood standards system building.

Table 1-1 Legal Framework for Blood Management

	Scheduled	Non-remunerated Blood Donation	Common Blood Establishment	Special Blood Establishment	Clinical Use of Blood	Plasma Center
Law	*Blood Donation Law of the People's Republic of China (1998)*					
Regulation	*Detailed rules or measures for the implementation of the Blood Donation Law of the People's Republic of China promulgated by provinces, autonomous regions and municipalities directly under the Central Government*					*Regulations on the Management of Blood Products (Revised 2016)*
Measures			*Measures for the Management of Blood Establishments (2017)*		*Measures for the Management of Clinical Use of Blood at Medical Institutions (2012)*	*Measures for the Management of Plasma Centers (2008)*
Standards			*Basic Standards for Blood Establishments (2000)*	*Management Measures for Umbilical Cord Blood Hematopoietic Stem Cell Banks (Trial) (1999)*	*Technical Specifications for Clinical Blood Transfusion (2000)*	*Basic Standards for Plasma Centers (2000)*
			Quality Management Practices for Blood Establishments (2006)	*Technical Specifications for Umbilical Cord Blood Hematopoietic Stem Cell Banks (Trial) (2002)*	*Quality Control Indicators for Clinical Use of Blood (2019 Edition) (2019)*	*Quality Management Practices for Plasma Centers (2006)*
	Guiding Principles for Setting up and Planning of Blood Establishments (2013)					

Continued

Scheduled	Non-remunerated Blood Donation	Common Blood Establishment	Special Blood Establishment	Clinical Use of Blood	Plasma Center
		Quality Management Practices for Blood Establishment Laboratories (2006)			Technical and Operational Procedures for Plasma Centers (2011 Version) (2011)
		Implementation Plan for Overall Promotion of Nucleic Acid Testing in Blood Establishments (2013-2015) (2013)			Notice on Plasma Center Management Related Issues (2012)
		Technical and Operational Procedures for Blood Establishments (2019)			Opinions on Promoting the Sound Development of Plasma Centers (2016)
		Notice on Promoting Non-remunerated Blood Donation (2019)			

Table 1-2　Blood Standards

Type	Name of Standard
National Standards	*Health Examination Requirements for Blood Donors* (GB 18467—2011)
	Quality Requirements for Whole Blood and Constituent Blood (GB 18469—2012)
Industrial Standards	*Commonly Used Terms for Blood Transfusion Medicine* (WS/T 203—2001)
	Blood Donation Site Configuration Requirements (WS/T 401—2012)
	Blood Storage Requirements (WS 399—2012)
	Blood Transportation Requirements (WS/T 400—2012)
	Guide for Monitoring the Quality of Whole and Constituent Blood (WS/T 550—2017)
	Guidelines for Classification of Adverse Reactions to Blood Donation (WS/T 551—2017)
	Guidelines for the Prevention and Management of Vasovagal Responses Associated with Blood Donation (WS/T 595—2018)
	Blood Transfusion in Internal Medicine (WS/T 622—2018)
	Whole Blood and Component Blood Use (WS/T 623—2018)
	Classification of Reactions to Blood Transfusion (WS/T 624—2018)

Chapter Two   Mechanism of Non-remunerated Blood Donation

I. Enhanced coordination mechanism of non-remunerated blood donation

In November 2019, 11 ministries and departments including the NHC released the *Notice on Promoting Non-remunerated Blood Donation* (2019, No. 21) to further promote the long-term mechanism of non-remunerated blood donation and its coordination to further consolidate the landscape featuring government leadership, departmental collaboration and universal participation in non-remunerated blood donation. Provinces, autonomous regions and municipalities directly under the central government, on the basis of their implementation of the *Blood Donation Law of the People's Republic of China*, focused more on government responsibilities. Provinces including Tianjin, Hebei, Nei Mongol, Liaoning, Jiangsu, Jiangxi, Henan, Guizhou and Gansu had put together provincial leading groups of non-remunerated blood donation, presided over by the competent vice governor. Held once or twice every year, the leading group deploys non-remunerated blood donation arrangements. Anhui, Hainan, Henan, Jiangsu, Jiangxi, Liaoning, Shanghai, Tianjin, Xinjiang, Ningxia, Zhejiang, Hebei, Kunming of Yunnan and some Sichuan cities integrated non-remunerated blood donation into the initiative of promoting intellectual and moral qualities. Guizhou, Henan, Hainan, Jiangsu, Zhejiang, Liaoning,

Ningxia and Tianjin incorporated non-remunerated blood donation into the government's performance targets.

II. Strengthened service system for blood establishments

1. Improving practitioner skills

In 2019, a total of 36,300 persons (36,307) were employed in blood establishments across the country, 800 fewer than in 2018, or 2.16% lower. Compared with 2018, an increase of staff with bachelor degree and above (Figure 1-1) was observed with an increase of 1.89 percentage points. Among them, the increase of staff with bachelor degree was 1.62%, that of staff with master's degree was 0.24%, and that of staff with doctoral degree was 0.03%. The number of personnel with junior college degree or below is decreasing year by year, showcasing an improving educational background. In 2019, health technicians accounted for 73.43% of the practitioners in blood establishments nationwide, a percentage similar to that in 2018 (Figure 1-2). The number of registered nurses increased by 1.17% compared with 2018, and the proportion of licensed (assistant) physicians, laboratory personnel and other health personnel decreased by 0.59%, 0.39% and 0.19% respectively over 2018. Among practitioners

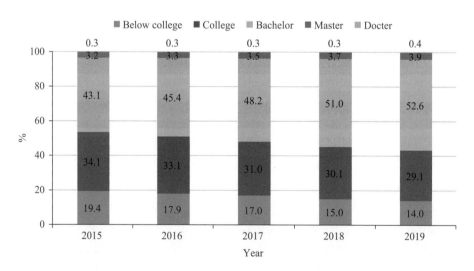

Figure 1-1   Educational background of blood establishment staff in China from 2015 to 2019

in blood establishments, an increase of the proportion of those with intermediate and senior professional titles had been observed in 2019 (Figure 1-3). Among them, the proportion of intermediate title increased by 0.32% and that of senior title increased by 0.49%.

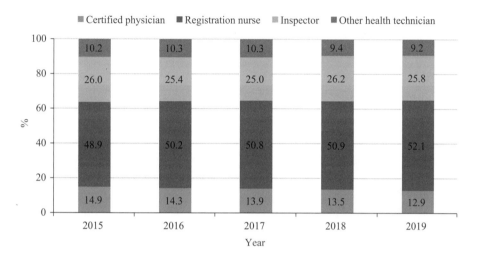

Figure 1-2   The composition of blood establishment staff in China from 2015 to 2019

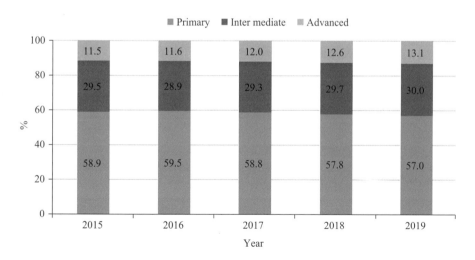

Figure 1-3   The proportion of professional titles of blood establishment staff in China from 2015 to 2019

2. Enhanced blood establishment infrastructure

In 2019, blood establishments nationwide covered a total area of 2.12 million square meters with a total construction area of 2.05 million square meters (Figure 1-4). The overall scale could accommodate the functional needs required of blood establishments. Meanwhile, the number of infrastructures such as fixed blood collection sites, blood collection vehicles and blood delivery vehicles in China was still on the rise (Figure 1-5).

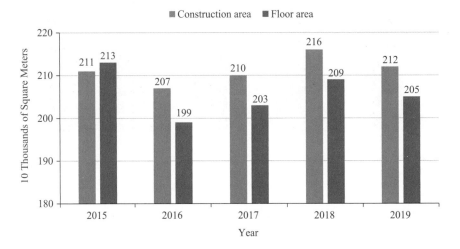

Figure 1-4   Land use of blood establishments in China from 2015 to 2019

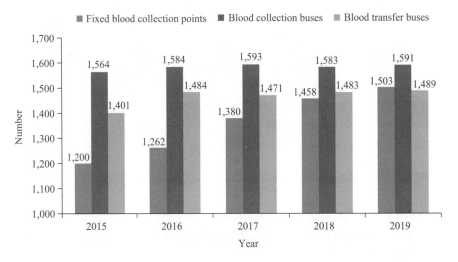

Figure 1-5   Status of fixed blood collection sites, blood collection vehicles and blood delivery vehicles in China's blood establishments from 2015 to 2019

The number of fixed blood collection sites increased by 45 compared with 2018, up 3.09%. The number of blood collection vehicles increased by 8 compared with 2018, up 0.51%. The number of blood delivery vehicles increased by 6 compared with 2018, up 0.40%.

3. Strengthened capability in blood management information

The national blood management information system was officially launched to collect real-time data on non-remunerated blood donation nationwide, with improved blood information management standards in provinces. Most provinces in China had established blood management information systems covering the entire province. Networking between blood establishments had been generally realized within the jurisdiction, and in some cities, networking between blood establishments and hospitals had been realized, making the whole process of blood collection, preparation, storage, transportation and clinical use safer and more controllable. Such provinces as Anhui, Guizhou, Hainan, Henan, Hunan, Jiangsu, Jiangxi, Shanghai, Tianjin, Zhejiang and Hebei among others had gradually built a provincially unified platform of cost reduction and exemption for blood expenses, forming a one-stop reduction mechanism primarily supported by medical institution's reduction and supplemented by network reduction for blood expenses incurred on non-remunerated blood donors and their relatives.

Progress was also made in regional information networking. As of the time when the report was prepared, networking in the Yangtze River Delta and the Beijing-Tianjin-Hebei Region was on the track to maturity. To integrate blood information networks in the Yangtze River Delta, a special meeting was held on August 16, 2019 in Hangzhou on the collective shielding and protection of blood donors during the interval period in the Yangtze River Delta blood collection and supply institutions. An information sharing network model was set up for blood donors during the interval period in this region. Zhejiang Blood Center took the lead in formulating basic data sets and interface specifications for information sharing and outlined the content entries in shared data. At present, the information sharing system for in-interval blood donors in blood collection and supply institutions in the Yangtze River Delta and for unqualified blood donors in Zhejiang Province has been completed. As a leading institution, Hebei Provincial Blood Center played an important role in promoting blood information networking in the Beijing-Tianjin-Hebei region, establishing a blood donor file sharing database for non-local reduction and exemption of blood expense, blood regulation, screening of unqualified blood donors, and sharing of resources of blood donors with rare blood types. These measures provided valuable practical experience for promoting regional blood information sharing in China.

III. Strengthened support for blood emergency

In 2019, China's health administrative departments at all levels had made innovations in blood emergency support and constantly optimized blood emergency support plans. Provinces and municipalities including Sichuan, Guizhou, Hainan, Henan, Jiangsu, Jiangxi, Liaoning, Nei Mongol, Shanghai, Tianjin and Hebei formulated blood emergency safeguard mechanisms. Provinces and municipalities including Anhui, Henan, Sichuan, Yunnan, Hainan, Hunan, Jiangsu, Liaoning, Nei Mongol, Ningxia, Shanghai, Tianjin, Xinjiang, Yunnan and Zhejiang integrated emergency management and blood regulation into their provincial blood management information system for coordination and unified management. Among them, the General Office of Hebei Provincial Government issued *Hebei Province Blood Emergency Plan*, which explicitly established a blood emergency safeguard system featuring hierarchical responsibility and territorial management. Emergency teams have been set up in various localities, and teams of group blood donor, constituent blood donors and rare blood donors had been formed. Government departments and public institutions at all levels should conduct research were required to gain a clear understanding of the number of healthy and appropriate aged staff members, set up emergency teams for non-remunerated blood donation based on participant's own will to respond swiftly to the call and participate in non-remunerated blood donation in case of emergencies or periodic blood shortage. Shanxi province had signed agreements on emergency blood donation with a number of institutions and groups, carried out physical examination for employees, and established an effective backup mobile blood bank for emergency use. As of the time, non-remunerated blood donation emergency teams in Shanxi province had over 18,000 team members, offering guarantee for clinical emergency blood use. Shandong province had set up three emergency blood banks: The provincial health system blood bank of good will, the mobile blood bank of blood establishment staff, and the Rh negative rare blood bank, as well as three emergency teams: The team of non-remunerated blood donation volunteers, the 110 blood donation team of college students, and the emergency team of machine platelet collection. A provincial blood emergency regulation system had been formed to strengthen the synergy between different regions in the province and realize real-time management of blood inventory and emergency vehicles. Jiangsu province had coordinated with the civil aviation departments to offer fast access to ensure blood regulation and aid to Xizang.

IV. Improved incentive mechanism for non-remunerated blood donation

Regions in China have stepped up their efforts in innovating the incentive mechanism of non-remunerated blood donation. Aided by legislative development, the reward for non-remunerated blood donation had been enriched with varied forms of reward for non-remunerated blood donation. Jiangsu and Zhejiang took the lead in proposing the three-exemption policy when revising their local legislation, which was very well received. In addition, Beijing had tried to introduce an insurance system to offer accident insurance to blood donors, whereas some cities in Zhejiang implemented the point-based settlement policy. Xiamen of Fujian province, had included non-remunerated blood donation in its "egret rating system". Citizens with a high egret rating can enjoy such "privileges" as deposit-free library borrowing and bike sharing services. The implementation of these specific measures had greatly promoted the sustained progress of non-remunerated blood donation in the region.

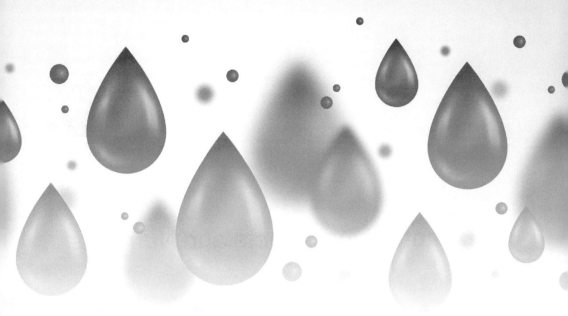

Section Two

Promotion of Non-remunerated Blood Donation

Chapter One   Facts and Numbers

I. Growing number of non-remunerated blood donations

A coordinated non-remunerated blood donation mode comprised of individuals and groups had been gradually formed in China. A total of 11.101 million non-remunerated donations had been observed in the country, an increase of 4.0% over 2018. Among them, 9.938 million were whole blood donations by individuals, an increase of 3.1% over 2018; together with 1.164 million platelet donations by individuals, an increase of 11.9% over 2018 (Table 2-1).

Table 2-1   The number and growth of voluntary non-remunerated
blood donation by individuals from 2015 to 2019

Year	Blood Donation / 10,000 Donations	Growth Rate/ %	Whole Blood Donation/ 10,000 Donations	Growth Rate/%	Platelet Donation/ 10,000 Donations	Growth Rate/ %
2015	961.3	—	881.9	−1.7	79.4	—
2016	1 013.1	5.4	927.6	5.2	85.5	7.7
2017	1 049.4	3.6	957.0	3.2	92.4	8.1
2018	1 067.6	1.7	963.6	0.7	104.0	12.5
2019	1 110.1	4.0	993.8	3.1	116.4	11.9

The proportion of non-remunerated group blood donation increased from 27.2% in 2018 to 27.6% in 2019 (Figure 2-1).

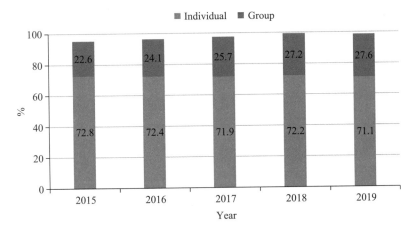

Figure 2-1   Proportion of voluntary non-remunerated donation by individuals and groups from 2015 to 2019

In 2019, voluntary non-remunerated blood donations nationwide reached 4.319 million, an increase of 7.2% over 2018. Among them, whole blood donation was 4.279 million, an increase of 7.2% over 2018 and platelet donation was 40000, an increase of 10.3% over 2018 (Table 2-2).

Table 2-2   The number and growth of voluntary non-remunerated blood donation by groups in China from 2015 to 2019

Year	Blood Donation/ 10,000 Donations	Growth Rate/%	Whole Blood Donation / 10,000 Donations	Growth Rate/%	Platelet Donation / 10,000 Donations	Growth Rate/%
2015	298.5	11.3	296.0	11.3	2.6	3.1
2016	337.2	13.0	334.5	13.0	2.7	4.8
2017	375.2	11.2	372.3	11.3	2.8	5.5
2018	402.7	7.4	399.1	7.2	3.6	25.8
2019	431.9	7.2	427.9	7.2	4.0	10.3

II. Progress towards balanced gender distribution of non-remunerated blood donors

The gender distribution of non-remunerated blood donors in China is gaining progress towards balance, with increasing share of female donors year by year (Figure 2-2). In 2019, women accounted for 37.6% of non-remunerated blood donors, up 0.5% from 2018. The gender distribution of non-remunerated blood donors was getting more balanced.

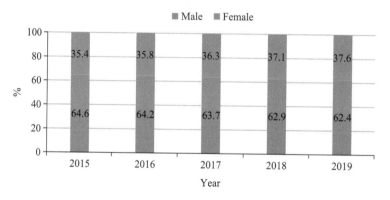

Figure 2-2   The gender distribution of non-remunerated blood donors from 2015 to 2019

III. Balanced age distribution of non-remunerated blood donors

Non-remunerated blood donors mainly aged between 18 and 45 years. In 2019, non-remunerated blood donors aged 18 to 44 accounted for around 77.0% of the total. There were around 890,000 non-remunerated blood donors above the age of 55 (Figure 2-3) from 2015 to 2019. There had been an increase of age for the non-remunerated blood donation population in China.

IV. Improving educational background of non-remunerated blood donors

The educational level of non-remunerated blood donors in China was on the rise in 2019. Non-remunerated blood donors were mainly comprised of junior high, senior high and junior college graduates. The proportion of blood donors with bachelor's degree increased from 19.8% in 2018 to 20.6% in 2019, and the proportion of primary, junior and senior high graduates blood donors showed a decreasing trend year by year (Figure 2-4).

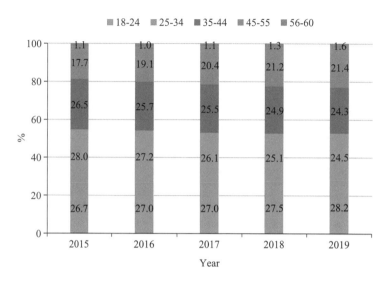

Figure 2-3   The age distribution of non-remunerated blood donors from 2015 to 2019

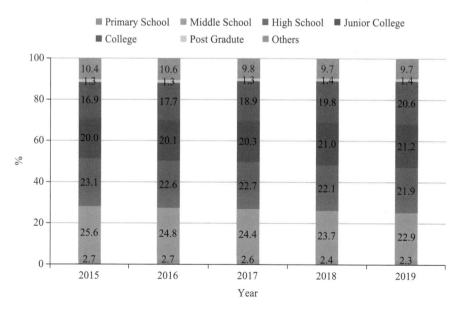

Figure 2-4   Educational backgrounds of blood donors from 2015 to 2019

V. Increased number of blood donation by college students year by year

Non-remunerated blood donors cover a wide range of professions including students, staff members, farmers, workers, medical personnel, civil servants, teachers, soldiers and others (i.e. freelancers). In 2019, the number of blood donation by college students accounted for 17.0% of the total number of donations, an increase of 0.7 percentage points compared with 2018, showing an upward trend year by year (Figure 2-5). The next step would be advancing the recruitment of non-remunerated blood donation to achieve donor diversity.

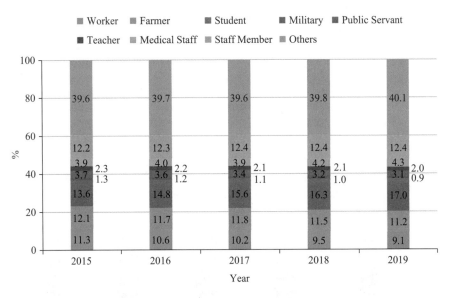

Figure 2-5   The proportion of non-remunerated blood donors in different professions from 2015 to 2019

VI. Increased per thousand population blood donation rate year by year

China's blood donation rate reached 11.2 per 1,000 people in 2019. In view of trend annually, the blood donation rate per thousand population in China increased year by year from 2015 to 2019, with an increase of 0.1 percentage point in 2019 compared with 2018 (Figure 2-6), further indicating that China's blood safety had been gradually strengthening.

VII. Decreased confidential withdrawal of blood

Confidential withdrawal of blood refers to the situation when, due to

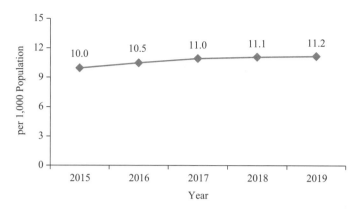

Figure 2-6   Blood donation rate per 1,000 population from 2015 to 2019

a donor's high-risk behavior that might have contaminated the donated blood, the blood service is informed after donation not to use the donated blood for clinical purposes. In accordance with the regulations, the national blood service shall, on the basis of protecting the privacy of the donor, label the blood as unqualified confidential blood. In 2019, the total volume of confidentially withdrawn blood in China was 3,757.7U, down 29.1% over 2018 (Figure 2-7).

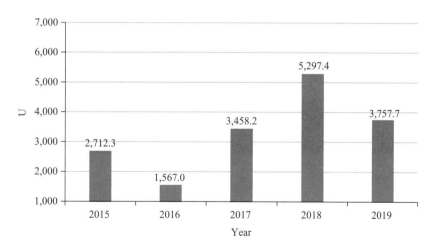

Figure 2-7   Volume of confidentially withdrawn blood from 2015 to 2019

VIII. Lowered ineligibility rate in blood screening

In 2019, the national blood screening ineligibility rate was 8.8%, down 0.2 percentage points over 2018 (Figure 2-8).

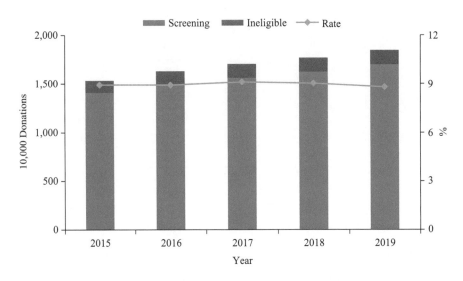

Figure 2-8   Ineligible blood in screening from 2015 to 2019

In 2019, alanine aminotransferase (ALT) was the main ineligible item that failed blood screening, accounting for 54.4%, down 2.1 percentage points from 2018. Hepatitis B surface antigen (HBsAg) took a share of 8.5%, down 1.2% over 2018, and hemoglobin (Hb) accounted for 14.4%, up 1.5 percentage points over 2018 (Figure 2-9).

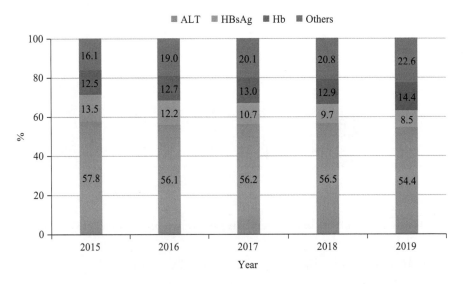

Figure 2-9   The ineligible items and their proportion in blood screening from 2015 to 2019

Chapter Two   Public Awareness of Non-remunerated Blood Donation

I. Diverse publicity campaigns for blood donation

The National Health Commission of China, the Red Cross Society of China and the Health Bureau of the Logistics and Support Department of the Central Military Commission jointly issued the 16th World Blood Donor Day promotional posters focusing on blood donation and safety of blood transfusion. China's ambassadors of non-remunerated blood donation, with their 30-second thematic video ad and print campaign, highlighted the theme of "safe blood for everyone".

Provinces, autonomous regions and municipalities directly under the central government had organized a variety of activities around the theme. With the help of media platforms including the Internet, television, radio, WeChat official accounts, positive energy was flowing among social members and tributes and gratitude were paid to the selfless blood donor community. Tianjin had created a new trend of blood donation promotion. The media made special reporting arrangements for broadcasting in fixed time periods and layouts, so as to create an all-round, multi-dimensional blood donation promotional network with varied forms of TV, radio, newspaper, website, WeChat and street scenes. Heilongjiang province had established a new blood donation mode of "blood donation month of medical personnel" in summer, "blood donation month for government departments and institutions" in autumn, "blood donation season for college students" in winter, and "blood donation period for groups and organizations" during New Year's Day and Chinese New Year. Shanghai recruited over 300 non-remunerated blood donors and staff from blood service to jointly participate in the MV of "My Motherland" with blood donation as its theme. The MV was screened on the Xuexi APP, Healthy China WeChat public account and some bus station advertisement slots in the city. Anhui province shot a promotional video entitled "Twenty Years' Endeavor, A Journey of Love, Devotion and Glory" and a documentary on the information system and practice of blood management. Kunming Blood Center of Yunnan and the Provincial Blood Transfusion Association jointly produced Yunnan's first non-profit micro film on blood donation — "Lifesaving Heroes", which won the excellent work award at the 7th Asian Micro Film Festival and the award of excellent drama work at the 4th Healthy China Micro Video Competition.

II. Continued commendation of non-remunerated blood donation

The Shanghai blood donation commendation conference 2019 was held in the Shanghai International Convention Center on June 13, the city's national and Shanghai blood donation awards winners were honored, with more than 700 individuals and representatives from organizations and competent leaders attended the conference. Shandong's six departments jointly launched the province's non-remunerated blood donation commendation conference, 465 organizations and 31,790 individuals were honored and officially recognized to promote selflessness and high morality of non-remunerated blood donation among the general public.

III. Direct reduction or exemption of clinical use of blood expenses for non-remunerated blood donors

The National Health Commission issued the *NHC General Office's Notice on Direct Reduction or Exemption of Clinical Use of Blood Expenses for Non-Remunerated Blood Donors* (hereinafter referred to as "The Notice"). The Notice required the relevant parties, keep in mind of donor-centered service, to fully put in place non-renumerated donor information connectivity between blood service and medical institutions in demand and the new reduction model primarily supported by medical institution and supplemented by online application. By the end of January 2020, Beijing, Hebei, Shanghai, Jiangsu, Zhejiang, Anhui, Jiangxi, Shandong, Henan, Hubei, Hunan, Guangdong, Hainan, Sichuan and Yunnan provinces had fully implemented the direct reduction and exemption of blood use expenses for non-remunerated blood donors and their relatives in hospitals located in their provinces.

Hebei province issued *Hebei Provincial Health Commission's Notice on Advancing Direct Reduction and Exemption of Blood Use Expenses for Non-Remunerated Blood Donors* to upgrade the province's Blood Expense Immediate Reimbursement of Blood Expenses for further simplifying blood expense reduction procedures, cutting review materials, optimizing workflow to provide more convenient and swift blood expense reduction and exemption services. Henan province issued the *Implementation Agenda for the Direct Reduction of Clinical Blood Expenses for Non-remunerated Blood Donors in Henan Province*, establishing a one-stop mode of reduction and exemption of blood expenses for the region's non-renumerated blood donors and their relatives, supported primarily by medical institutions and supplemented with online reduction and exemption. Guangdong had established a unified information platform, completed the transformation of the government service cloud server and the database of the medical treatment information system for public health emergencies, and took the lead in launching the direct reduction and exemption of clinical use of blood expenses for non-remunerated blood donors in several areas of Guangzhou. Shanghai municipality had set up a working group to formulate the agenda of direct reduction and exemption of clinical use of blood expenses for non-remunerated blood donors, analyzed the implementation steps of the policy of free blood use for non-remunerated blood donors as well as the qualifying rules of "direct exemption", and formulated the rules of out-of-pocket expenses and forward transfer of funds.

IV. Three types of exemptions for non-remunerated blood donors
Several provinces, such as Hebei, Hainan, Jiangsu and Zhejiang,

had implemented the policy of three types of exemption for individuals who have been commended for non-remunerated blood donation by the country. The three types of exemption included exemption of admission tickets for government-funded or -sponsored parks and scenic spots, exemption of general outpatient consultation charges in public medical institutions and the exemption of tickets for urban public transportations.

The Hainan Special Economic Zone's Regulation on Non-remunerated Blood Donation was also implemented in 2019. Article 16 of the regulation stipulates that donors who had non-remunerated donation records in the zone and had been awarded National Award for Non-remunerated Blood Donation, National Gratuitous Award for Non-remunerated Hematopoietic Stem Cell Donation and National Lifetime Honor for Voluntary Service in Non-remunerated Blood Donation were entitled to the above three types of exemptions in the zone. Hebei province issued Notice on Implementing Articles on Three Types of Exemption in Non-remunerated Blood Donation in Hebei Province, and jointly issued the Notice on Better Implement the "Three Exemption" Policy for Non-remunerated Blood Donation with the Provincial Red Cross Society to make sure that the "Three Exemptions" policy was appropriately followed through by relevant departments.

V. Long-term mechanisms in support of non-remunerated blood donation

For this end, Beijing had established an information monitoring and scheduling mechanism involving health administrative departments at the municipal and district levels, blood collection and supply institutions and 29 major hospitals for blood use. Under the leadership of the General Office of the Shandong Provincial Government, 12 departments jointly established a joint conference system of blood donation at the provincial level, and all 17 municipalities in the province established leading groups of non-remunerated blood donation for the timely reporting of blood donation progress. Henan, with communications with the Henan Provincial Office of Cultural Advancement, integrated non-remunerated blood donation into the Henan Model Organization Assessment System. Sichuan, together with several ministries and commissions, issued the

Notice on the Establishment of the Inter-department Joint Conference System for Non-remunerated Blood Donation in Sichuan Province, establishing a coordinated and synergized structure with government as the leader based on multi-department cooperation and universal participation of the public.

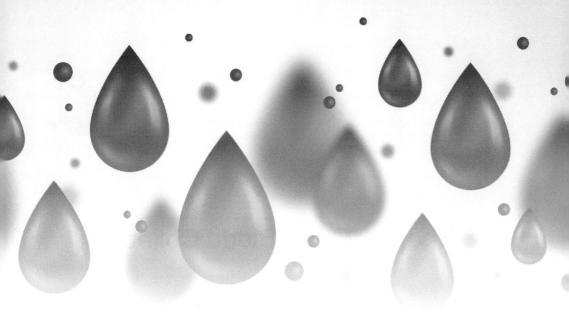

Section Three

Blood Establishments and Quality Assurance

Chapter One   Blood Collection

Since 1998, the amount of non-remunerated blood donation in China has been increasing year by year, maintaining a sustained growth for 21 years. In 2019, 15.623 million blood donations were collected, an increase of 5.6% over 2018. Among them, 14.4 million whole blood donations and 1.22 million platelets donations were collected, an increase of 5.1% and 12.1% over 2018, respectively (Figure 3-1).

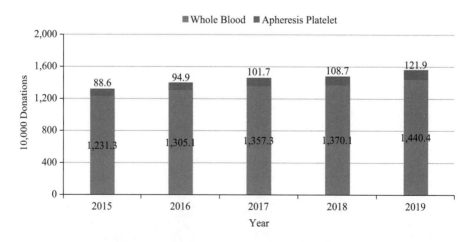

Figure 3-1   Blood donations collected from 2015 to 2019

In the past five years, the total amount of blood collected nationwide has continued to rise. In 2019, 24.45 million units of whole blood were collected, an increase of 5.0% over 2018. The platelets for 2.04 million treatments were collected, an increase of 14.8% over 2018 (Figure 3-2).

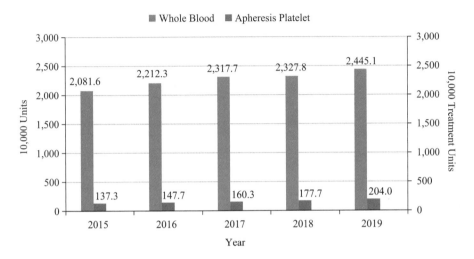

Figure 3-2   Blood donations in units and for treatments from 2015 to 2019

According to the *Blood Donation Law of the People's Republic of China*, a donor usually donates 200ml of blood at each donation, with the maximum volume being 400ml. With more blood donation campaigns in recent years, people's understanding and support of blood donation has been increasing. As a result, the proportions of 300ml and 400ml donations saw sustained growth. While the proportion of 200ml blood donation in 2019 was 18.1%, which was 0.3% lower than that in 2018, the average volume of the whole blood donation was 340.6ml, which was 0.2ml higher than that in 2018 (Figure 3-3).

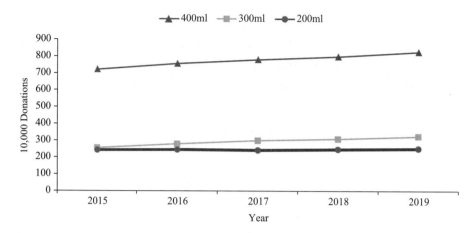

Figure 3-3   Ratios of whole blood donations at 200ml / 300ml / 400ml from 2015 to 2019

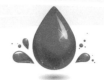

Chapter Two   Preparation and Supply of Blood Components

Transfusion of blood components is an important indicator that measures the development of blood transfusion technology of a hospital, a region or a country. Since the promulgation of the *Blood Donation Law of the People's Republic of China* in 1998, much progress has been made in the cause of blood transfusion, with the proportion of blood component transfusion growing year by year. In 2019, the separation rate of blood components in China's blood establishments reached 99.9%.

I. Increased supply of blood components

At present, the main types of supply of blood components for clinical use in China include whole blood, red blood cells, platelets and plasma.

Whole blood. The whole blood released by national blood establishments was 32,000 units in 2019, 24.4% less than that in 2018 (Figure 3-4).

Red blood cells. These mainly include red blood cells in additive solution, washed red blood cells, thawed red blood cells, leukocyte-reduced red blood cells and irradiated red blood cells. In 2019, 24.472 million units of red blood cells were supplied by the blood establishments, an increase of 8.2% over 2018. Leukocytes reduced red blood cells accounted for the largest proportion (68%), followed by red blood cells in additive solution (26.5%) (Figure 3-5).

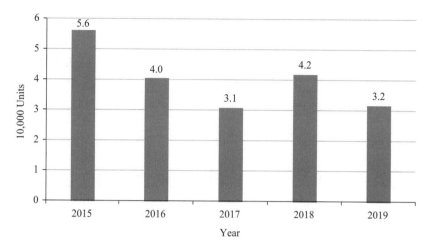

Figure 3-4　Volume of clinical supply of whole blood from 2015 to 2019

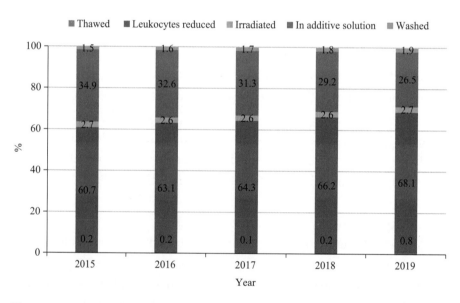

Figure 3-5　Ratios of the clinical supply of red blood cells by category from 2015 to 2019

Platelets. These include apheresis platelets and platelet concentrates. From 2015 to 2019, the apheresis platelet supply was abundant and increased year by year. In 2019, 2.039 million units of apheresis platelets were collected from blood establishments in China, a growth of 14.6% over 2018. On the other hand, the platelet concentrate supply was small.

In 2019, 501,000 units of platelet concentrates were collected from blood establishments in China, a decrease of 4.4% over 2018 (Figure 3-6).

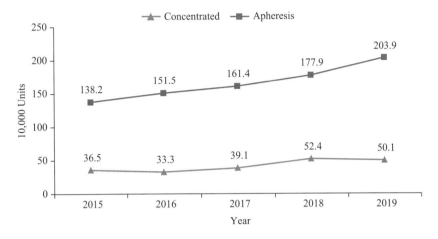

Figure 3-6   Volume of clinical supply of apheresis platelets and platelet concentrates from 2015 to 2019

Plasma. It mainly includes fresh frozen plasma, frozen plasma and virally inactive plasma. In 2019, 24.224 million units of plasma components were issued from the blood establishments in China, an increase of 13.6% over 2018 (Figure 3-7).

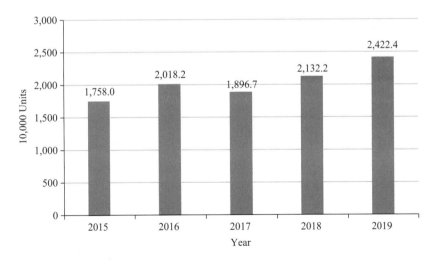

Figure 3-7   Volume of clinical supply of plasma from 2015 to 2019

The utilization rate of formed elements is one of the important indexes to evaluate the overall utilization and quality management of blood at the blood establishments. Since 2016, China has seen an upward trend in the utilization rate of formed elements. The utilization rate in 2019 was 102.0%, 0.1 percentage points lower than that of 2018 (Figure 3-8).

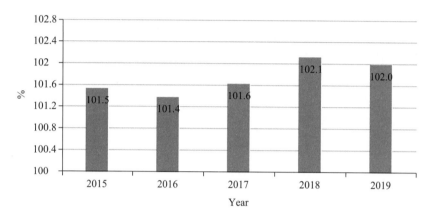

Figure 3-8　The utilization rates of formed elements from 2015 to 2019

II. Balanced blood supply and collection through effective (re) distribution

China has established and implemented a coordinated blood supply mechanism, improving the blood distribution and inventory management system, and collaborating supply in key areas and at important time points. China redistributed 3.143 million units of blood components throughout the year of 2019. With such a mechanism, different regions struck a good balance between blood collection and supply and guaranteed an effective and steady supply. From 2015 to 2019, the proportions of blood component inventories stabilized, maintaining a good balance across different inventories (Figure 3-9).

III. Improved management of discarded blood

Discarded blood is divided into two cases: test-based discarding and physical discarding. Test-based discarded blood refers to unqualified blood from laboratory testing and confidentially withdrawn blood from donors engaging in high-risk behavior, whereas physically discarded blood refers

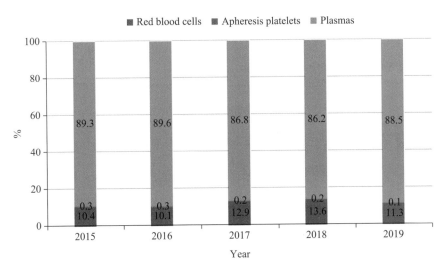

Figure 3-9   Ratios of blood component inventories from 2015 to 2019

to rejected blood products due to abnormal appearance (chylaemia, blood bag damage, etc.) and otherwise qualified blood products rejected for being past their shelf life. Physically discarded blood is one of the indexes for assessing the management of blood establishments.

In 2019, the volume of physically discarded blood was 1.741 million units, an increase of 15.1% over 2018. In addition, the ratio of physically discarded blood was 3.2%, 0.1 percentage point higher than that of 2018 (Figure 3-10).

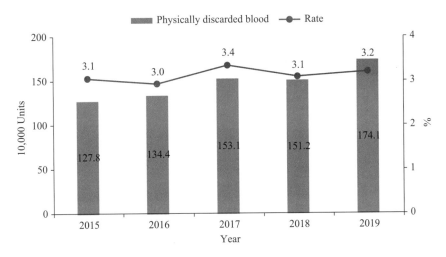

Figure 3-10   Ratios of physically discarded blood from 2015 to 2019

In 2019, the main cause for physically discarded blood was abnormal appearances, accounted for 90.4% of all physical discarding, 6 percentage points lower than that of 2018 (Figure 3-11).

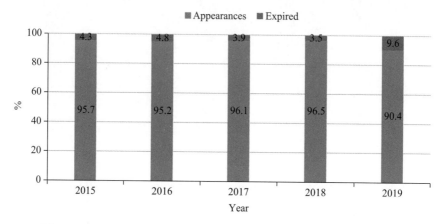

Figure 3-11 Physically discarded blood by cause from 2015 to 2019

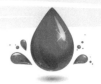

Chapter Three   Blood Testing

Blood tests at the laboratories of the blood establishments aim at screening of transfusion-related pathogens, including alanine aminotransferase (ALT), hepatitis B virus surface antigen (HBsAg), hepatitis C virus antibody (anti-HCV), human immunodeficiency virus antigen and antibody (anti-HIV), Treponema pallidum antibody (anti-TP) and the nucleic acid test (NAT) of HBV, HCV and HIV. With enhanced pre-donation screening technology and capacity-building of the blood establishments in China, the rate of unqualified blood samples from laboratory tests has been declining. In 2019, the unqualified rate was 2.1%, similar to that in 2018 (Figure 3-12).

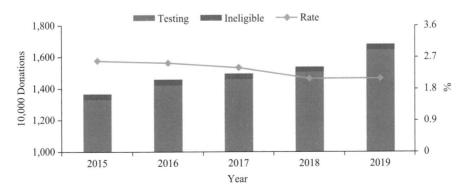

Figure 3-12   Rates of unqualified blood samples at the blood establishments from 2015 to 2019

In 2019, ALT was the primary cause of ineligible blood donations at the blood establishments, accounting for 44.6% of the total. The second cause was HBsAg, accounting for 19.2% (Figure 3-13).

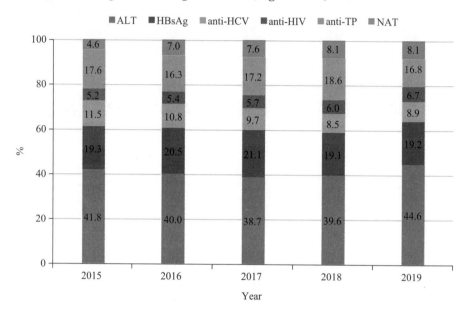

Figure 3-13   Ratios of ineligible blood donations by different screening items from 2015 to 2019

The annual trends of the tested items showed that the disqualification rate due to ALT increased slightly in 2019 (Figure 3-14).

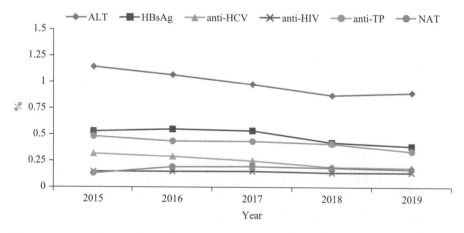

Figure 3-14   Disqualification rates by different tested items at the blood establishments from 2015 to 2019

Chapter Four Quality Assessment

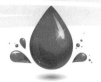

External quality assessment (EQA), also known as external quality assurance, is an important part of an internationally recognized laboratory quality management system. The way an EQA program works is that an organizer sends the test samples to the participating laboratories on a regular basis, the participating labs carry out the tests within the specified time and return the results. The organizer then analyzes the test results of each laboratory, and gives a quality assessment report according to the pre-defined standards. The EQA not only evaluates the testing quality of the participating labs, but makes an overall analysis on the comparability and accuracy of the results across different laboratories. Through the independent and systematic evaluation of the labs' testing capacity, the EQA schemes promotes the blood testing quality of all labs. Therefore, the regulators attach great importance to the important role that the EQA programs play in ensuring blood safety through quality assurance of the laboratories.

With the development of the blood test technology and the increase of test items, the EQA system for laboratories of Chinese blood establishments has developed from scratch to full-fledged programs. The reporting methods has transported from printed letters to electronic reports. A comprehensive laboratory quality assessment system has been established for the blood service. At present, the Clinical Testing Center of the National Health Commission (hereinafter referred to CTC) includes 11 items in four EQA programs when evaluating the laboratories of blood collection and supply institutions, covering all the routine tests. The system has contributed positively to blood safety in China. The items included in each EQA program are different due to different quality assessment schemes selected by the blood establishments, hospitals, plasmapheresis establishments and manufacturers of reagents and biological products.

In 2019, the number of blood establishments participating in the CTC EQA programs was roughly the same as that in 2018. The test items of some blood banks and collection sites only included serological and blood group tests. And the nucleic acid tests of some regional blood banks were contracted to third-party institutions. The schemes selected by different blood establishments in the EQA programs were not identical (Table 3-1).

Table 3-1   Basic situation of the EQA programs for
laboratories of the blood establishments

EQA Programs	Tested Items	2018 Blood establishments/ No.	2019 Blood establishments/ No.
Blood Tests for Infectious Disease	ALT, HBsAg, anti-HCV, anti-HIV, anti-TP	358	357
Tests for Blood Group	ABO, Rh (D)	350	348
Nucleic Acid Tests	HBV DNA, HCV RNA, HIV RNA	308	312
Test for HTLV Antibody	HTLV Antibody	76	81

Blood Tests for Infectious Disease. In 2019, a total of 357 blood establishments participated in the EQA schemes for infectious diseases. Among them, 351 establishments had qualified results, with a qualification rate of 98.3%. There were six unqualified establishments due to late submission of lab reports. In addition, the detection rate of HBsAg was significantly improved. Although the EQA samples were more difficult in 2019, only one laboratory missed the detection. This indicated that the previous feedback had been noted, with necessary rectification measures implemented.

NAT. All laboratories participating in the NAT EQA were qualified, with scores above 80 points. There were 279 laboratories with 100% accurate results, accounting for more than 90% of the total. The result was significantly better than that in 2018.

Blood Group Tests. In 2019, 336 laboratories were qualified during the two EQAs. Three laboratories failed to report the results on time once, and 9 laboratories had test errors. As a result, a total of 12 laboratories failed the blood group tests in 2019, and 3 of them failed because of late submission of lab reports.

In 2019, 206 blood establishments from 29 provinces (as well as autonomous regions and municipalities directly under the central government) participated in the EQA programs, including 27 blood centers and 179 regional blood banks, which was only 60% of the total. Problems were found for some blood establishments, including insufficient equipment, poor maintenance and unstable reagent performance. These problems were difficult to find through the EQA, but could be revealed by comparison of lab quality indicators. Therefore, each establishment should pay attention to the reporting of comparable quality indicators.

Chapter Five   Quality Assurance

Health administrative departments at all levels attach great importance to blood quality and safety. They have strengthened the quality assurance system and carried out blood safety technical verification for blood establishments and clinical use of blood. On this basis, local stakeholders have also boosted blood quality and safety management through information sharing and innovative mechanisms.

I. Stringent technical verification for blood safety

The National Health Commission organized technical verification for blood safety in 21 provinces (as well as autonomous regions and municipalities directly under the central government) in 2019. The inspection covered compliance with blood safety laws and regulations, quality management specifications and technical operation procedures. On-site inspection and interaction were arranged for blood establishments, plasmapheresis establishments and medical institutions. All local stakeholders were required to learn from isolated problems found during the inspection and initiate rectification. With improved blood quality management at all levels, blood safety for clinical use was enhanced as well.

II. Enforcement of and compliance with blood safety laws and regulations

All provinces (as well as autonomous regions and municipalities directly under the central government) focus on improving the capacity for blood safety and supply. Through the annual verification of the working conditions of blood establishments and plasmapheresis establishments, and the technical review for license renewal, compliance with relevant national laws and regulations were ensured. At the same time, provincial, municipal and county regulators comprehensively check the blood establishments, medical institutions and apheresis establishments for law enforcement and supervision according to the frequency stipulated by the state (once at the provincial level, twice at the municipal level and four times at the county level). Combined with special supervision schemes, the standard of practice of the blood collection and supply system was raised, with better assessment and stricter inspection of the key links for blood safety than before. Hidden threats for blood safety were discovered and uprooted in a timely manner.

III. Better response measures for blood safety

All provinces (as well as autonomous regions and municipalities directly under the central government) regularly carry out internal audits and external quality assessments to improve laboratory testing capacity, standard and quality assurance. In 2019, Beijing formulated a local standard for *Technical Specifications of Blood for Clinical Use at the Medical Institutions*, and revised the quality assurance documents such as *Quality Assessment Standards of Blood Transfusion Departments or Blood Banks of Beijing Medical Institutions* (300 points) and *Quality Assessment Indices of Blood Transfusion Departments or Blood Banks of Beijing Medical Institutions*. As a result, the quality assurance system of blood for clinical use was enhanced. Some provinces and cities adopted innovative measures for remote monitoring, daily and sample checks to ensure the quality of blood products. All plasmapheresis establishments in Heilongjiang Province upgraded their video monitoring system to carry out whole-process and real-time supervision of the plasmapheresis facilities. Provincial and municipal stakeholders strengthened the training of practitioners. At the various links of blood collection and supply, various forms of blood safety training courses were delivered. The blood emergency plans were made to classify different emergency events, clarify the organization and responsibilities of emergency supply, and organize regular drills to ensure quick response in case of emergency.

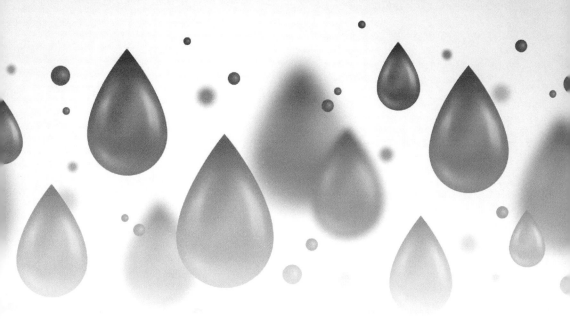

Section Four

Clinical Use of Blood

With accelerated industrialization, urbanization and population aging, the working and life styles of the Chinese people and the associated disease spectrum are evolving. Under the Healthy China 2030 strategy, health administrative departments, guided by the philosophy of science-based, coordinated, equitable, accessible, safe and effective development, focused on the promotion of law-based governance, supply, safety and rational use of blood. Management of the clinical use of blood has been strengthened from various perspectives, including evidence-based rationality and safety of use.

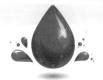

Chapter One   Managing Clinical Use of Blood

I. Deepened system-building for clinical use of blood

In NHC's 2019 revision of *Measures for the Management of Clinical Use of Blood by Medical Institutions*, articles on mutual-assisted blood donation in the original version of the Measures were repealed. Given the advantages that medical institutions have in promoting health education, more efforts were made by them to strengthen public awareness of voluntary non-remunerated blood donation, and rational and safe use of blood for patient health. In the same year, the NHC issued *Quality Control Indicators for Clinical Use of Blood* (2019, 620) (2019), which specified ten quality control indicators for clinical use of blood as well as their definitions, significance and calculation formula. The regulation was not only a nation-level step to improve clinical use of blood for diagnosis and treatment at medical institutions, but a guiding protocol for standardized and rational use of blood. It contributed to developing consistency, capacity and professionalism in blood transfusion.

At the provincial level, the health administrative departments of Beijing, Hebei, Shaanxi, Gansu and Hainan, among others, formulated or revised the quality control indicators and standards for the blood transfusion departments at medical institutions or blood establishments within their own jurisdictions. The health administrative departments of Beijing, Liaoning, Henan and other provinces or municipalities also formulated or revised the technical specifications, management framework and operational guidelines for clinical use of blood at the medical institutions. The overall institutional building for standardized management of clinical use of blood management was enhanced.

II. Strengthened quality control of clinical use of blood

The National Health Commission took the annual national blood safety technical inspection as a starting point to boost supervision and regulation of blood safety in all provinces. Under the framework of the national blood safety technical inspection, provincial health departments conducted supervision and inspection on clinical use of blood at their own medical institutions. For instance, Shanghai carried out performance assessment of its medical institutions, focusing on the management framework for clinical use of blood, and simulated blood transfusion inspection at hospitals with modest use of blood. Emphasis was placed on the practical improvements of clinical use of blood at medical institutions via differentiated examinations. For hospitals with relatively small amount of blood use (or inconsistent need for blood transfusion), a thematic examination named "transfusion of a bag of blood" was implemented to simulate pre-transfusion preparation, blood collection and delivery, transfusion, follow-ups and other operation-oriented inspections. The purpose of inspection at all levels was to find out the problems and verify the corresponding rectification, so as to promote evidence-based clinical use of blood.

Under the guidance of provincial health departments, provincial quality control centers for clinical use of blood leveraged their professional skills in regulating appropriate clinical use of blood at medical institutions under their jurisdiction. Nei Mongol and Guizhou encouraged the set-up of transfusion committees at the primary care providers and transfusion departments at Grade II (secondary) or above hospitals to oversee clinical use of blood.

III. Enhanced training on the clinical use of blood

In 2019, provincial health departments and quality control centers for the clinical use of blood held varied training courses to raise the awareness of clinical medical workers for blood safety and rational use of blood. The training covered a wide range of topics including management of the clinical use of blood, transfusion skills, relevant laws and regulations, pre-job training and practitioner assessment. Special trainings were offered to directors of quality control centers for the clinical use of blood, directors and core technicians of blood transfusion departments. Seminars and academic salons were organized for young researchers of blood transfusion. Some provinces (as well as autonomous regions and municipalities directly under the central government) also held clinical blood transfusion skill competitions to improve professionalism and expertise of the technicians.

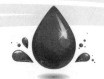

Chapter Two　Rational Use of Blood

According to the data from the Hospital Quality Monitoring System (HQMS) of the National Health Commission, there was consistent inpatient blood use of the ten surgeries indicated in the component blood transfusion records in the NHC-affiliated and non-affiliated Grade III (or tertiary) hospitals. Among the ten indicated surgeries, there was no significant difference in blood use for cesarean section between NHC-affiliated and non-affiliated hospitals. However, there was significantly more blood use for cardiopulmonary surpassed surgery and abdominal aortic aneurysm surgery at non-affiliated hospitals than those at NHC-affiliated hospitals (Figure 4-1-Figure 4-3).

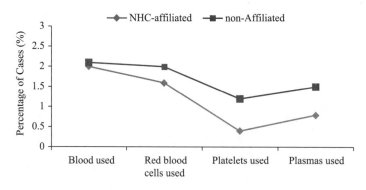

Figure 4-1　Institutional comparison of blood use for cesarean section

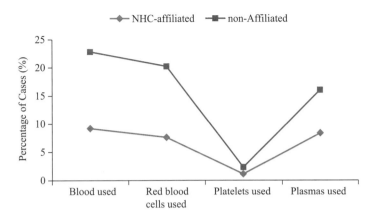

Figure 4-2   Institutional comparison of blood use for cardiopulmonary bypass surgery

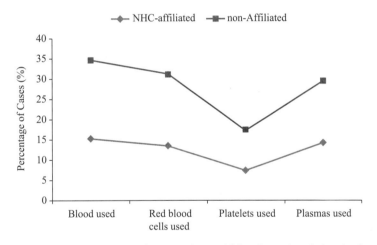

Figure 4-3   Institutional comparison of blood use for abdominal aortic aneurysm surgery

Data revealed that among the patients with blood use records, the vast majorities were allogeneic blood transfusion, with autologous transfusion accounting for only 2.2% of all transfusions. For eight out of the ten indicated surgeries, the amount of autologous blood used by NHC-affiliated hospitals was higher than that in non-affiliated hospitals.

By introducing new technologies and applications, blood use at medical institutions was managed to a more rational level. The Fuwai Hospital of the Chinese Academy of Medical Sciences (Fuwai Hospital) adopted innovative practices such as preoperative anemia drug therapy, extracorporeal circulation surgery for the preventative use of tranexamic acid, extracorporeal circulation pipeline to reduce prefilling volume, minimal blood sampling to limit diagnostic blood loss, and thromboelastography for treatment of bleeding patients. Ever since the implementation of Fuwai's multidisciplinary blood management eleven years ago, the average use of red blood cells and plasma decreased by 68.6% and 80.1% respectively, though the number of cardiovascular surgeries increased by nearly 95%. For six consecutive years, the amount of autologous transfusion (intraoperative recovery autologous transfusion) exceeded the amount of allogeneic transfusion. In 2019, more than 70% of cardiovascular surgeries did not involve blood transfusion. The rate of blood transfusion in adult cardiovascular surgeries dropped to 23.9%, 12.7% and 10.5% respectively. Meanwhile, postoperative hospitalization, surgical mortality and complications were substantially reduced. The rate of cardiac surgery without blood transfusion dropped to one of the world's lowest levels. Blood use of Fuwai Hospital in the past five years is shown in Figure 4-4 to Figure 4-8.

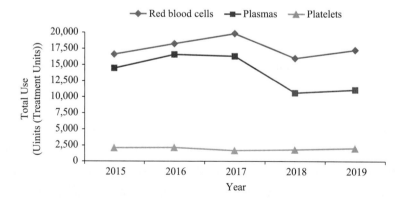

Figure 4-4   Blood use at Fuwai Hospital in the past five years

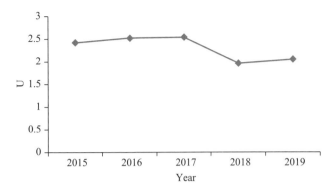

Figure 4-5   Average blood use per operation at Fuwai Hospital in the past five years

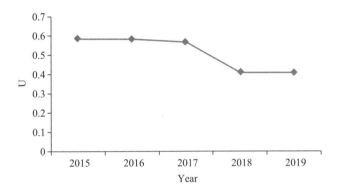

Figure 4-6   Per capita blood use of discharged patients at Fuwai Hospital in the past five years

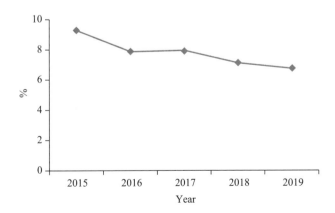

Figure 4-7   Proportion of patients receiving blood transfusion at Fuwai Hospital in the past five years

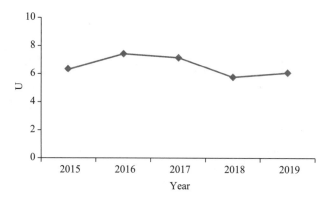

Figure 4-8   Per capita blood use by transfused patients at Fuwai Hospital in the past five years

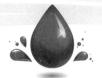

Chapter Three   Active Hemovigilance

As a special form of medicine, it is inevitable for blood usage to encounter adverse reactions though its purpose is to save lives. Compared with other medicines, adverse reactions (ADR) to transfusion usually occurs with more frequency and severity. Reducing ADRs is a concrete measure to reduce irrational blood use and safeguard patient health. ADR monitoring and surveillance for blood transfusion forms the foundation of the blood safety warning system. It is the most effective and cost-efficient measure to ensure sustainable blood safety in China. Therefore, the NHC incorporated the indicator of number of ADR cases reported per 1,000 transfusion into *Quality Control Indicators for Clinical Use of Blood* (2019 Edition) to give better guidance in establishing an ADR reporting system for blood transfusion.

According to data from the Key Laboratory of Adverse Reaction in Blood Transfusion of the Chinese Academy of Medical Sciences, a total of 1,933 cases of adverse reactions to blood transfusion had been reported by 188 hospitals in 29 provinces since the ADR data management system was officially launched on May 1, 2018.

Of the 1,933 cases, 29 were identified to be unrelated to adverse reaction to transfusion, 229 were identified as 'possible', 'suspected to be', or 'uncertain'. The rest 1,675 cases were identified as "certain" or "likely" to be associated with transfusion adverse events.

Main types of adverse reactions included allergic reactions, 74.27%, and non-hemolytic febrile reactions, 23.28% (Figure 4-9).

The main blood components involved in transfusion ADR in China were apheresis platelets, 32.60%, red blood cell additive solution, 29.97%, and plasma, 34.69% (Figure 4-10).

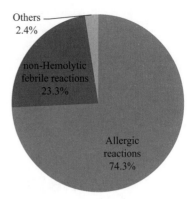

Figure 4-9   Types of adverse reactions to transfusion

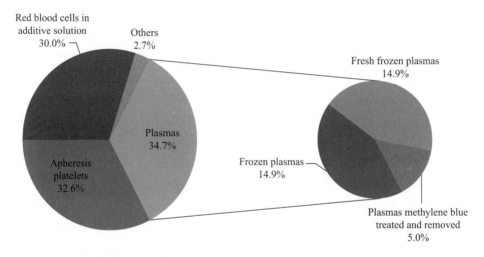

Figure 4-10   Main blood components involved in adverse reactions to transfusion

Among all allergic reactions, 94.45% of allergic reactions were mild cases and 5.55% were serious ones.

From 2018 to 2019, a total of 1,244 cases of allergic reactions were reported, accounting for around 3/4 (74.27%) of all ADR cases in the year. The blood components involved in allergic reactions were mostly plasma, apheresis platelets and red blood cell additive solutions (Figure 4-11).

A total of 390 cases of non-hemolytic fever were reported from 2018 to 2019, accounting for about a quarter (23.28%) of all ADR cases of the year, second only to allergic reactions. The blood components causing

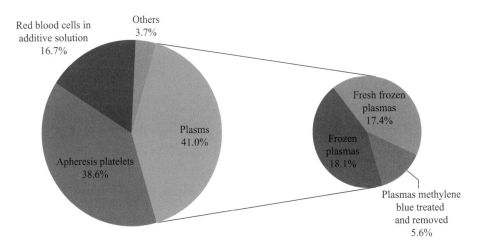

Figure 4-11　Blood components involved in allergic reactions

non-hemolytic fever reaction were predominantly red blood cell additive solution (271 cases), followed by apheresis platelets (55 cases) and plasma (60 cases) (Figure 4-12).

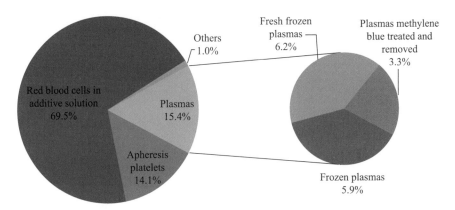

Figure 4-12　Blood components involved in non-hemolytic fever reactions

There had only one incidence of adverse reaction caused by autologous blood transfusion which was indeed allergic reaction. Therefore, by increasing the proportion of autologous transfusion, adverse reactions may well be reduced.

Hemovigilance forms the foundation of blood safety warning. As an effective tool and approach to improving blood safety, it is attracting more and more attention from administrative departments and medical institutions. As an integral part of the blood management system, hemovigilance is not only intended for monitoring adverse reactions to blood transfusion, but also for finding out the causes of these adverse reactions and weak links in blood safety. Addressing these problems can enhance our ability to maintain blood safety, making sure that an effective hemovigilance system is in place. Staying vigilant of risks and problems and earnestly implementing early warning, prevention and control are some of the most important measures to ensure rational and safe use of blood in clinical settings of China.

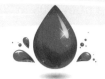

Chapter Four Quality Assessment

The external quality assessment (EQA) of transfusion compatibility is an external quality assurance program launched by the Clinical Testing Center of the National Health Commission, which authenticates, verifies and confirms the capability of blood transfusion departments of medical institutions or blood establishments to carry out blood testing for clinical transfusion compatibility. By revealing and comparing existing problems, it offers a path for assessing and cross-referencing the testing results of the participating laboratories to improve their testing capability. As such, it acts as one of the bedrocks for safe and appropriate clinical use of blood.

The 2019 EQA programs included five test items: ABO forward typing, ABO reverse typing, the RhD blood group, antibody screening and cross-matching. All the items were reviewed according to the accreditation criteria for proficiency testing providers (ISO/IEC 17043) by China National Accreditation Service for Conformity Assessment (CNAS). The institutions participated in the EQAs mainly included blood transfusion departments and laboratory departments of medical institutions, laboratories of blood collection and supply institutions and reagent manufacturers, as well as the blood transfusion departments and blood collection and supply institutions of some military medical institutions. In 2008, there were only 200 participating institutions. The number surged from 2008 to 2014, registering an average growth rate of 39%. The number of participating institutions gradually plateaued with an average annual growth rate of 7% from 2015 to 2019.

In 2019, the number of participating institutions reached 2,314. Among them, 1,218 were Grade III (or tertiary) Level A hospitals, in which 1,160 were civilian hospitals and 58 were military hospitals; 309 were Grade III Level B hospitals, in which 304 were civilian hospitals and 5 were military hospitals; 516 were Grade II (or secondary) Level A hospitals, including 511 civilian hospitals and 5 military hospitals; and 51 Grade II Level B hospitals, all of which were civilian hospitals. Then there were another 154 hospitals, including 148 civilian hospitals and 6 military hospitals, that did not specify their grading, and 66 non-hospital institutions. At least 13 provincial departments of quality assessment participated in the EQA programs with over 4,000 participating institutions which were predominantly Grade II medical institutions in their respective province. See Figure 4-13 for the specific numbers of participating laboratories from 2008 to 2019 in the country. There were 2,314 participating institutions from 31 Chinese provinces, municipalities and autonomous regions in 2019, excluding Chinese Taiwan, Macao SAR and Hong Kong SAR. Please refer to Figure 4-14 for the specific distribution of participating institutions nationwide from 2015 to 2019.

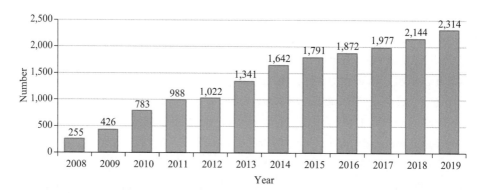

Figure 4-13　Number of institutions participating in the EQAs of blood transfusion compatibility testing from 2008 to 2019

Note: The above statistics applied for all EQAs.

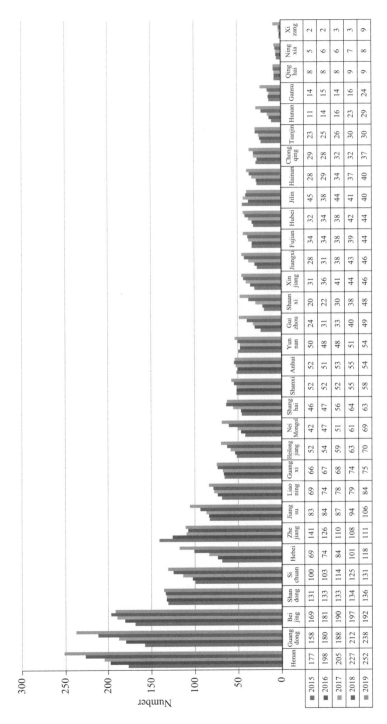

Figure 4-14   Regional distribution of institutions participating in EQAs from 2015 to 2019

Three rounds of quality assessment were carried out in the EQAs of blood transfusion compatibility during the year, which included the test items of ABO forward typing, ABO reverse typing, RhD blood group, antibody screening and cross-matching. See Table 4-1 for the complete 2019 assessment results of the five test items according to the types of participating institutions. The participating institutions were qualified only if all five EQA items were qualified. The results of each item are shown from Figure 4-15 to Figure 4-19. The qualification rate of participating institutions from different provinces, municipalities and autonomous regions from 2015 to 2019 are presented in Figure 4-20.

Table 4-1　Results of the five EQA items by the type of participating institutions

Type of participating institution	Total participating institutions/No.	Number of institutions with 5 qualified items/No.	Proportion of institutions with 5 qualified items/%
Grade III Level A	1,218	1,003	82.35
Grade III Level B	309	230	74.43
Grade II Level A	516	356	68.99
Grade II Level B	51	30	58.82
Unreported	154	113	73.38
Other	66	52	78.79
Total	2,314	1,784	

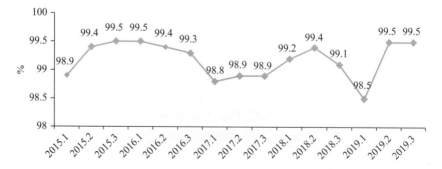

Figure 4-15　EQA results of ABO forward typing from 2015 to 2019
Note: 2015.1 represents the first batch of EQAs in 2015, and the rest are similar.

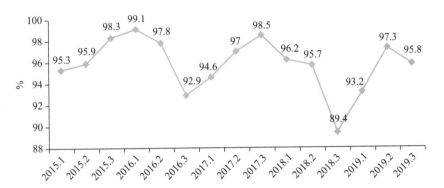

Figure 4-16   EQA results of ABO reverse typing from 2015 to 2019

Note: 2015.1 represents the first batch of EQAs in 2015, and the rest are similar.

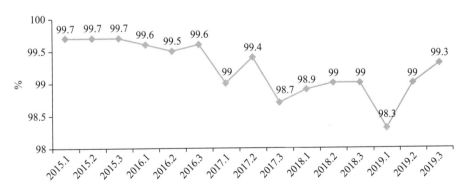

Figure 4-17   EQA results of RhD blood group from 2015 to 2019

Note: 2015.1 represents the first batch of EQAs in 2015, and the rest are similar.

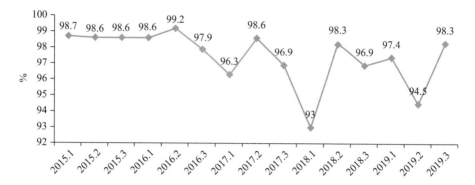

Figure 4-18　EQA results of antibody screening from 2015 to 2019
Note: 2015.1 represents the first batch of EQAs in 2015, and the rest are similar.

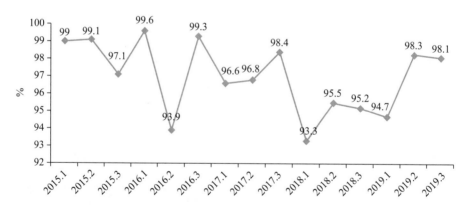

Figure 4-19　EQA results of cross-matching from 2015 to 2019
Note: 2015.1 represents the first batch of EQAs in 2015, and the rest are similar.

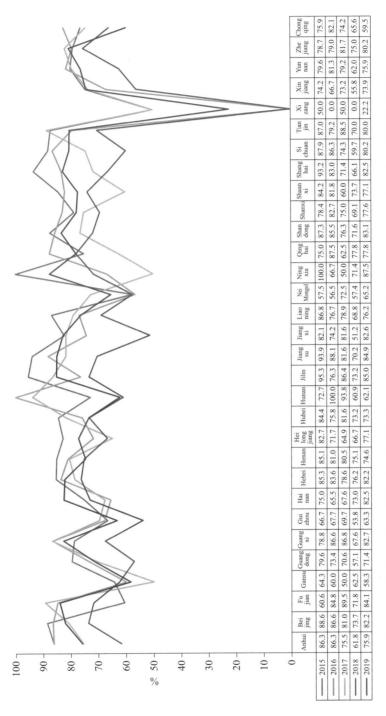

	Anhui	Bei jing	Fu jian	Gansu	Guang dong	Guang xi	Gui zhou	Hai nan	Hebei	Henan	Hei long jiang	Hubei	Hunan	Jilin	Jiang su	Jiang xi	Liao ning	Nei Mongol	Ning xia	Qing hai	Shan dong	Shanxi	Shaan xi	Shang hai	Si chuan	Tian jin	Xi zang	Xin jiang	Yun nan	Zhe jiang	Chong qing
2015	86.3	88.6	60.6	64.3	79.6	78.8	66.7	75.0	85.3	85.1	82.7	84.4	72.7	95.3	93.9	82.1	86.8	57.5	100.0	75.0	87.3	78.4	84.2	93.2	87.9	87.0	50.0	74.2	79.6	78.7	75.9
2016	86.3	86.6	84.8	60.0	73.4	86.6	67.7	65.5	83.6	81.0	71.7	75.8	100.0	76.3	88.1	74.2	76.7	56.5	66.7	87.5	85.5	81.8	81.8	83.0	86.3	79.2	0.0	66.7	81.3	79.0	82.1
2017	75.5	81.0	89.5	50.0	70.6	86.8	69.7	67.6	78.6	80.5	64.9	81.6	93.8	86.4	81.6	81.6	78.9	72.5	50.0	62.5	76.3	75.0	60.0	71.4	74.3	88.5	50.0	73.2	79.2	81.7	74.2
2018	61.8	73.7	71.8	62.5	57.1	67.6	53.8	73.0	76.2	75.1	66.7	73.2	60.9	73.2	70.2	51.2	68.8	57.4	71.4	77.8	71.6	69.1	73.7	66.1	59.7	70.0	0.0	55.8	62.0	75.0	65.6
2019	75.9	82.2	84.1	58.3	71.4	82.7	63.3	82.5	82.2	74.6	77.1	73.3	62.1	85.0	84.9	82.6	76.2	65.2	87.5	77.8	83.1	77.6	77.1	82.5	80.2	80.0	22.2	73.9	75.9	80.2	59.5

Figure 4-20   Rate of participating institutions with five qualified items across regions from 2015 to 2019

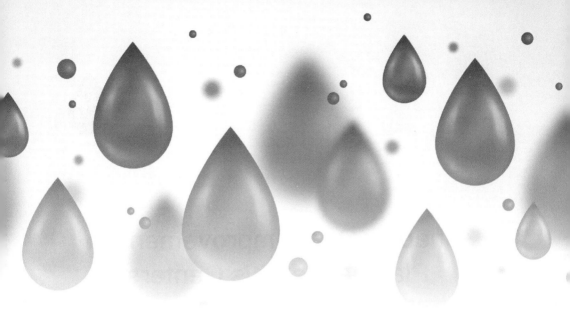

Section Five

Plasmapheresis Centers

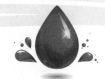

Chapter One   Improvement of Plasmapheresis Centers

I. Increasing Plasmapheresis Centers

In 2019, 26 provinces (as well as autonomous regions and municipalities directly under the central government) and the Xinjiang Production and Construction Corps had plasmapheresis centers in China. Among them, the Xinjiang Production and Construction Corps approved the establishment of their first plasmapheresis center. The total number of plasmapheresis centers in China increased from 182 in 2015 to 237 in 2019. The number of plasmapheresis centers in Sichuan, Guangdong and Guangxi accounted for 36.3% of the total (Figure 5-1).

II. Stronger information systems for plasmapheresis centers

In 2019, Zhejiang province developed a data collection and reporting system for plasmapheresis centers. The Blood Center of Zhejiang Province took the lead in formulating the specifications of data sharing via uniformed datasets and data interface. So far, the information sharing and vigilance systems for unqualified plasma and blood donors had been set up. According to the *Implementation Plan of Developing Blood Management Information System in Shanxi Province*, the information management system of all plasmapheresis centers should follow the unified coding standards

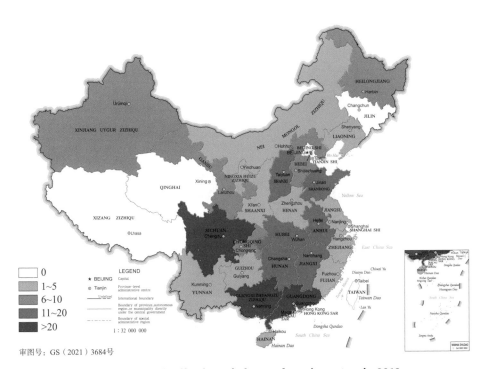

Figure 5-1　Distribution of plasmapheresis centers in 2019
(Remark: the data of this figure do not include HONG KONG SAR, MACAU SAR and TAIWAN Province.)

and procedure control system to harmonize data feeding within the provincial blood management information system. A supervisory platform for plasmapheresis centers was also established in Gansu, ushering in an era of information-based management of plasmapheresis centers for this region.

According to the survey results, 169 plasmapheresis centers supported by 19 blood products enterprises invested 24.271 million yuan in building or upgrading their information systems in 2019.

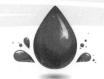

Chapter Two   Plasma Donors and Plasma Collection

I. Plasma Donors

Registered qualified plasma donors totaled 3.667 million with farmers as the main groups, accounting for 75% of the total donors, followed by other professions, 17% (Figure 5-2). According to the statistics of all provinces (as well as autonomous regions and Xinjiang Production and Construction Corps), the volume of raw plasma collected in 2019 increased by 13.6% compared with the previous year. 17 provinces (as well as autonomous regions and Xinjiang Production and Construction Corps) showed year-on-year growth. There were 25.654 million plasma donations in China in 2019. The largest source of raw plasma donations was Sichuan province, followed by Shandong and Guangxi provinces.

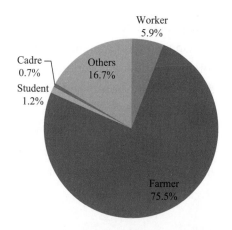

Figure 5-2   Ratio of qualified plasma donors by profession, 2019

II. Better services for plasma donors

According to the survey results, a total of 357.48 million yuan from 19 blood product enterprises was invested in improving the services for plasma donors. These included setting standards for services in plasmapheresis centers, publishing *Blood Collection and Supply Institutions Staff Manual*, upgrading the infrastructure, creating a better plasma-donating environment, providing donors and their families with discounts on blood products, paying regular visits to donors with gift bags, working with local governments on poverty alleviation for source regions and providing financially challenged donors with subsidies.

Chapter Three　Plasma Testing

I. Laboratory Testing

Plasmapheresis centers carried out laboratory testing in accordance with relevant requirements of the State. The tests at plasmapheresis centers mainly included ALT, HBsAg, hepatitis C virus antibody (anti-HCV), human immunodeficiency virus antibody (anti-HIV) and treponema pallidum antibody (anti-TP).

In 2019, the total number of failed laboratory plasma tests at plasmapheresis centers in China reached 33,000. The incidence of HBsAg non-conformities was the highest, accounting for 53% of the total (Figure 5-3). This

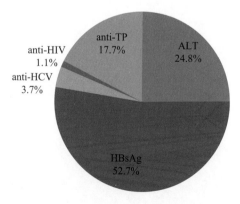

Figure 5-3　Ratio of ineligible plasma based on laboratory testing at plasmapheresis centers in China in 2019

was followed by ALT non-conformities, 25% of the total.

II. External Quality Assessment (EQA)

In 2019, 52 plasmapheresis centers participated in the EQA schemes of blood tests for infectious diseases, six more than that of 2018. All 52 plasmapheresis centers were qualified, with a qualification rate of 100%. In 2019, 117 plasmapheresis centers participated in various quality assessment schemes, doubling the number of 2018 (Figure 5-4).

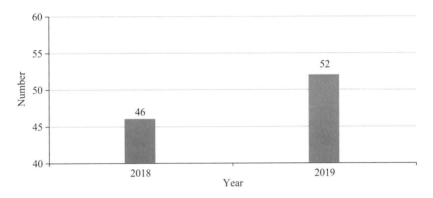

Figure 5-4   Number of plasmapheresis centers/ biological products factories participating in EQAs from 2018 to 2019

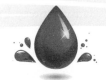

Chapter Four Quality Management and Supervision

Governments at all levels prioritized the quality management and supervision of plasmapheresis centers. The provincial health departments aimed at enhancing the supervision of plasmapheresis centers in their respective regions, forming inspection panels to engage in on-site inspections with much attention paid to the rectification of the issues.

Some provincial health departments formulated and introduced documentations on standardized management of local plasmapheresis centers. Jiangxi formulated the *Scoring System for Undesirable Operations at Plasmapheresis Centers in Jiangxi Province* (draft for comments) and the *Evaluation Criteria for On-Site Inspections of Plasmapheresis Centers in Jiangxi Province* (draft for comments), which were implemented in 2020. Guangdong drew up the *Working Guidelines for Administrative Examination and Approval of Plasmapheresis Centers* and a *Notice on Comprehensive Improvement of the Management of Plasmapheresis Centers in Guangdong Province* and the *Scoring System for Undesirable Operations at Plasmapheresis Institutions in Guangdong Province* (for Trial Implementation) to advance the management system of plasmapheresis centers.

With the backing of the blood information management platforms at provincial level, Zhejiang, Anhui, Hunan and Shaanxi provinces exercised remote and real-time administration on plasmapheresis centers to improve their management.

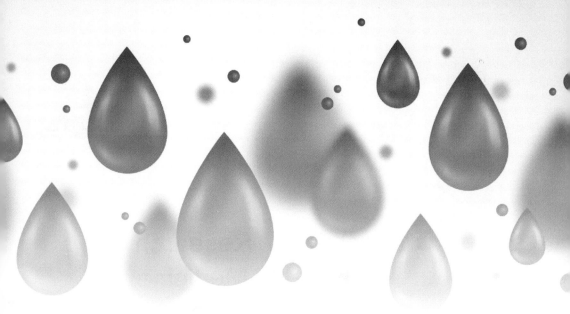

Section Six

Transfusion Medicine:
Research and Education

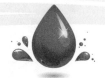

Chapter One   Research of Transfusion Medicine

I. Building research teams

In 2019, according to statistics from nineteen provincial blood centers, two municipalities with independent planning status (Dalian and Qingdao) and some research institutes, most blood centers had research scientists on their payrolls.

Among full-time researchers, 92% of them hold a bachelor's or higher degrees, which include 44% of them holding a bachelor's degree, accounting for the lion's share, 36% of them holding a master's degree and 12% having a doctoral degree and postdoctoral research background (Figure 6-1).

Among full-time researchers, the proportion of researchers with professional titles (intermediate and above) accounted for 75% of the total, with 16% of the researchers having full senior titles and 23% having associate senior titles (Figure 6-2).

II. Research projects

In 2019, according to incomplete statistics, six national scientific research projects were granted to blood researchers with a total of 1.34 million yuan in funds. Among them, scientists from the Blood Transfusion Research Institute of the Chinese Academy of Medical Sciences, the

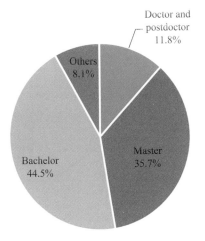
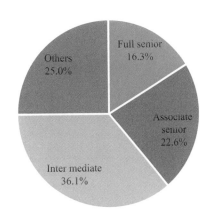

Figure 6-1   Distribution of the educational levels of full-time researchers

Figure 6-2   Distribution of professional titles of full-time researchers

Shanghai Blood Center, the Chengdu Blood Center and Zhejiang Blood Center won the scientific research grants from the National Natural Science Foundation.

Urumqi Blood Center's project on the follow-up of blood donors with HBV was funded by the National Health Commission's Programs for Natural Science Foundation for Young Scientists. Thirty-five provincial and ministerial level scientific research projects with a total funding of about 5.69 million yuan were also approved. These research grants focused on stem cell, clinical transfusion and decision-making model study, education and Institution-building and transfusion-transmitted diseases.

There were twelve ongoing national projects with a total funding of about 8 million yuan. The projects were mainly initiated by the Blood Transfusion Research Institute of the Chinese Academy of Medical Sciences and the Shanghai Blood Center, Zhejiang Blood Center and the No. Six Affiliated Hospital of Xinjiang Medical University. There were 43 provincial and ministerial level scientific ongoing research projects with a total funding of about 7 million yuan (Figure 6-3).

III. Scientific and technological achievements

According to incomplete statistics, a total of six national, provincial, ministerial and municipal (prefecture) scientific and technological awards

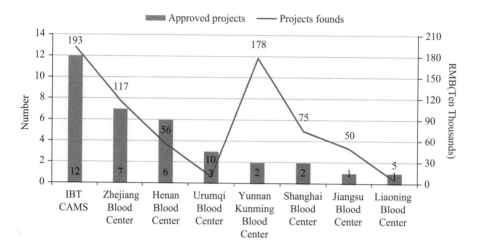

Figure 6-3 Top eight institutions by provincial and ministerial level project funds in 2019

were granted to the institutions in the blood transfusion industry. Among them, two scientific and technological awards were granted to the joint project on polymorphisms of ligand gene in KIR and HLA in nine minority ethnic groups of Yunnan Province investigated by Yunnan Kunming Municipal Blood Center and the Blood Transfusion Research Institute of the Chinese Academy of Medical Sciences.

The other four awards were granted to the Chinese Academy of Medical Sciences, Gansu Red Cross Blood Center, Dalian Blood Center and Qingdao Blood Center.

Twelve national invention patents and thirty-five patents on utility models were approved and authorized, mainly in the fields of detection method and diagnostic kit of Multiplex polymerase chain reaction of the genotype of human platelet, automated blood collection tube dryer, a method for content determination of sialic acid in IgG Fab and Fc fragments of IVIG and the Preparation Method of PBT that is anti-platelet adhesion and does not affect platelet function.

Seven national invention patents and thirty patents on utility models initiated by Qingdao Blood Center were approved and authorized, mainly in the fields of blood collection devices, solution diluters, blood bags and laboratory reagents (Figures 6-4, 6-5 and 6-6).

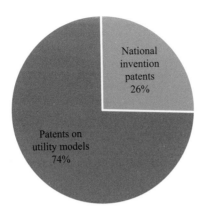

Figure 6-4   Types of patents that were approved and authorized

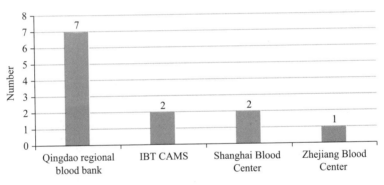

Figure 6-5   Institutions obtaining invention patents in 2019

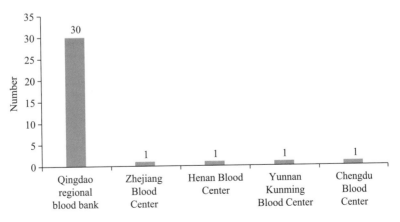

Figure 6-6   Institutions obtaining patents on utility models in 2019

IV. Research Papers

According to initial statistics, there were 80 SCI research papers published by Chinese researchers of transfusion medicine as the first author or corresponding author in 2019. Among those papers, the majority were published by researchers of the Institute of Blood Transfusion of the Chinese Academy of Medical Sciences (19 papers) with a cumulative impact factor of 55.89 points, followed by Zhejiang Blood Center (18 papers) with a cumulative impact factor of 50.4 points.

The Shanghai Blood Center published 12 research papers with a cumulative factor of 39 points. The published papers covered the areas of blood immunology, transfusion-transmissible agent and relevant testing and biochemistry. 107 articles were published in core Chinese academic journals, along with 239 articles published in non-core Chinese academic journals (Figures 6-7, 6-8 and 6-9).

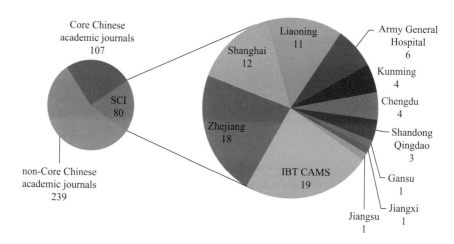

Figure 6-7   SCI research papers published by Chinese researchers of transfusion medicine

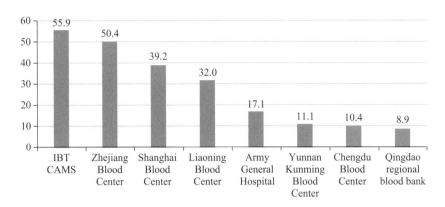

Figure 6-8   Top eight institutions by the total impact factor of SCI publications in 2019

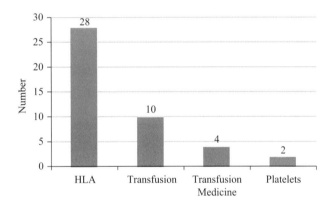

Figure 6-9   Top four SCI journals by the number of articles published in 2019

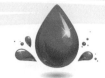

Chapter Two Continuing Education of Transfusion Medicine

In recent years, various blood collection and supply institutions and medical institutions with clinical use of blood have strengthened the management of continuing education and training of practitioners. Special panels were set up to be responsible for improving staff participation in continuing medical education. Targeted training plans and modules were formulated. The yearly promotion of employees became linked to their accumulated training points of that year. In 2019, a total of 53 national and provincial continuing education programs were offered, covering 5,740 trainees in more than 1,100 class hours. The training modules included laboratory biosafety and management, promotion of unpaid blood donation and recruitment of voluntary donors, management of clinical blood transfusion and blood testing, among others.

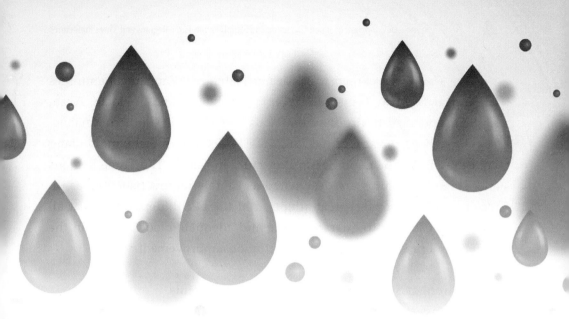

Section Seven

Development of Blood Collection and Supply in the Three Regions and Three Prefectures

The *Three Regions* refer to 1) Xizang Zizhiqu, 2) Zangzu communities in Qinghai, Sichuan, Gansu and Yunnan Provinces, and 3) Hotan, Aksu, Kashgar, and Kizilsu Kirgiz Autonomous Prefectures in southern Xinjiang. The *Three Prefectures* refer to Liangshan Prefecture in Sichuan, Nujiang Prefecture in Yunnan and Linxia Prefecture in Gansu. The Three Regions and Three Prefectures are designated as acutely impoverished areas. In recent years, under the great attention of the health departments at all levels, the capacity to guarantee safe and adequate blood supply in the regions and prefectures registered continuous improvement.

I. Stronger Support for the Blood Establishments

The investment in the construction of blood establishments in the Three Regions and Three Prefectures kept increasing, with the service systems constantly improving. By 2019, 24 blood centers had been established in the Three Regions and Three Prefectures. According to the survey data, the total amount of financial reources allocated to these five regional blood banks (Table 7-1) in 2019 was 24.205 million yuan, a six-fold growth from those of 2015 (Figure 7-1).

Table 7-1   Blood establishments in the Three Regions and Three Prefectures

Province	Name	Number of personnel/ People.	Actual on-duty personnel/ People.	Floor area/m^2
Qinghai	Yushu regional blood bank	8	8	1,000
Qinghai	Guoluo regional blood bank	8	7	960
Qinghai	Haibei regional blood bank	11	11	634
Xinjiang	Kizilsu Kirgiz regional blood bank	15	13	—
Sichuan	Ganzi regional blood bank	20	13	1,084

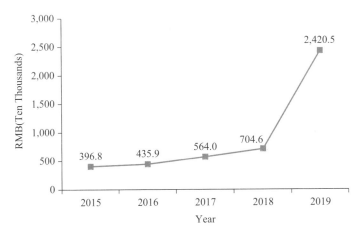

Figure 7-1   Amount of financial resources to blood establishments in the Three Regions and Three Prefectures in 2019

II. Improved Blood Collection Capacity

In 2019, the total number of blood donors at five regional blood banks was 5,005, and the total blood donation was 8,038 units, which increased by 37.8% and 42.8% respectively compared with those in 2015 (Figure 7-2). The proportion of individual voluntary non-remunerated blood donation was 89.6% (Figure 7-3). The total number of hospitals supplying blood increased from 31 to 40, and the longest blood supply distance increased from 1,152 km to 1,199.1 km (Figure 7-4).

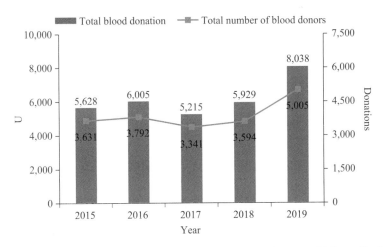

Figure 7-2   Donation at blood centers in the Three Regions and Three Prefectures from 2015 to 2019

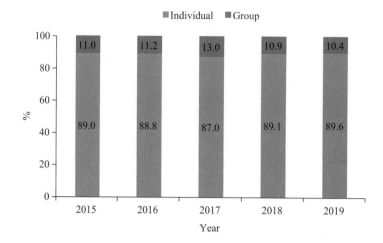

Figure 7-3 **Percentages of individual and group voluntary nonremunerated blood donation in the Three Regions and Three Prefectures from 2015 to 2019**

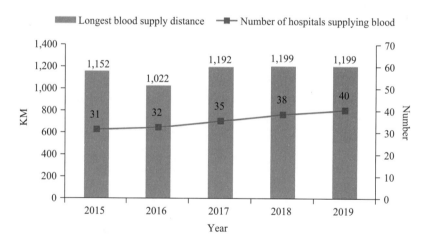

Figure 7-4 **Blood supply by blood centers and hospitals in the Three Regions and Three Prefectures from 2015 to 2019**

III. Enhanced blood supply capacity

At present, the main types of clinical blood supply at the five blood centers are whole blood, red blood cell components and plasma components, red blood cell component blood accounting for the highest proportion. Specifically, the whole blood supply in 2019 was merely 20.1 units, 84.9% lower than that in 2015 while 10,312.3 units and 7,411.5 units of red blood cell component blood and plasma component blood were issued respectively in 2019, 29.5% and 35.6% higher than those in 2015 (Figure 7-5).

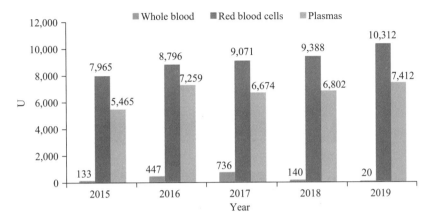

Figure 7-5   Clinical blood supply from blood centers in the Three Regions and Three Prefectures from 2015 to 2019

IV. Blood Screening

From 2015 to 2019, the rate of unqualified blood in the pre-donation blood screening at the 5 blood centers rose slightly from 6.1% to 6.8%, and this rate at blood screening laboratories after blood collection dropped from 5% to 3.7%, finally increasing to 6.4% (Figure 7-6).

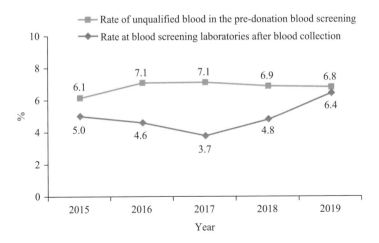

Figure 7-6   Blood screening at blood centers in the Three Regions and Three Prefectures from 2015 to 2019

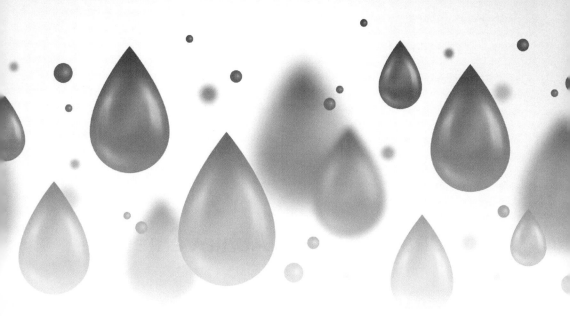

Section Eight

Future Prospects

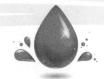

Chapter One   Achievements

Non-remunerated blood donation is a key social undertaking that has a direct bearing on people's health and safety, prioritized by the Community Party of China and the Chinese government. Since the implementation of the *Blood Donation Law of the People's Republic of China* in 1998, under the leadership and strong support of the Party committees, governments, and relevant departments at all levels, and with the active participation of the public, China established the system of non-remunerated donation in full swing, and the legal system of blood management and the service system of blood collection and supply in blood centers have been increasingly improved. In 2019, the total number of non-remunerated blood donors in China registered at 15.623 million, representing a year-on-year growth of 4.0%. The blood donation rate reached 11.2 per 1000 people. There is a sound non-remunerated blood donation system in China, which is well-managed for rational use of blood on an evidence-based manner and with powerful guarantees.

I. A long-term legal system of blood management

In 2019, the National Health Commission continued to adhere to "opening source, controlling expenditure, and ensuring safety", with the main orientation towards improving the law-based governance, blood supply, blood safety, and rational blood use. To constantly promote the legal system, it further updated relevant regulations and technical standards in the light of the *Blood Donation Law of the People's Republic of China, Measures for the Management of Blood Establishments*, and *Measures for the Management of Clinical Use of Blood at Medical Institutions*. It continued to strengthen the blood quality control system, facilitated technical procedures, standards, and specifications of blood centers and plasma centers, enhanced personnel training and assessment to elevate the quality of professional personnel, guided blood centers and plasma centers to establish the blood management quality control and sustained improvement system covering the whole process of blood collection and supply, and conducted regular internal auditing and EQA. As a result, blood quality management became increasingly better, and the rate of discarded blood and adverse events related to blood quality kept declining and remained at a low level.

II. An improved information system for blood management and services

China strengthened information-based management of blood safety and improved the information-based service. In 2019, China basically formed the blood management information system and provincial blood management information system, which covered all blood centers. Regional information-based management platforms were built in some regions, such as the Yangtze River Delta integrated blood information-based platform and the Beijing-Tianjin-Hebei blood information-based network. The shared database of blood donors' files was established to realize free reductions and exemptions for blood use in other places, blood distribution, the screening system of high-risk blood donors, resource sharing of blood donors with rare blood types, etc. Some provinces set up provincial-level platforms for free exemptions or fee reductions for blood use, forming a one-stop compensation model for blood transfusion expenses of voluntary non-remunerated blood donors and their relatives. The compensation was mainly cleared at medical institutions, and sometimes through online reimbursement. The service capacity and service level were enhanced thanks to information-based management.

III. Enhanced blood collection and supply capacity

China has built the efficient blood center service system with blood centers focusing on regional blood banks, and complemented by remote county-level blood banks, which covers urban and rural areas. In 2019, China further promoted the dynamic early warning and monitoring of blood inventory and the blood distribution mechanism that basically solved the challenge of seasonal, regional, and rare-type blood supply shortage faced by the world.

China reinforced technical procedures, standards, and specifications of blood centers of blood centers, promoted the information-based management, improved the whole process quality management system of blood collection and supply, established the screening system for high-risk blood donors and the cold chain management system for blood transportation and storage, and conducted regular internal auditing and EQA. As a result, the rate of discarded blood and adverse events related to blood quality kept declining and remained at a low level. China fully implemented the blood nucleic acid testing strategy, effectively shortened the "window period" of the human immunodeficiency virus (HIV), hepatitis B virus, and hepatitis C virus testing, and basically blocked the transmission of HIV and other key infectious diseases transmitted by blood transfusion.

By the end of 2019, China basically achieved full coverage of nucleic acid testing of raw plasma, which shows that China's blood safety has stepped onto a new stage.

IV. Strengthened technological support for blood safety

Clinical blood quality control centers have been established in various localities, with efforts made to improve the training, supervision, management, evaluation, and notification system of clinical use of blood, recognizing clinical use of blood as a key indicator of medical quality assessment. These local stakeholders promoted the understanding and experiences of clinical use of blood and standardized and rational use of blood. They strictly controlled indications of blood use, guided medical institutions to strengthen blood management for patients, popularized evidence-based blood transfusion strategies, promoted protective technologies such as autologous blood transfusion, and reduced intraoperative bleeding and adverse reactions during allogeneic blood transfusion.

In the past five years, the average blood consumption of discharged patients and operating table dropped by 20% and 30% respectively, and the proportion of autologous blood transfusion increased by 30%.

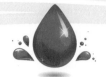

Chapter Two   Challenges

Blood supply and blood safety are the important foundation of clinical medicine and people's health. Since the implementation of the *Blood Donation Law of the People's Republic of China* 20 years ago, China's blood safety management level has seen rapid development; however, the traditional and new blood safety risks remain. With the building of the moderately prosperous society in all respects and the in-depth building of the "Healthy China", and the continuous improvement of the social demand for the capability to guarantee blood safety, blood safety is still encountering challenges.

I. The distribution of the blood establishments needs to be optimized.

There is insufficient investment in blood establishments at the primary level. The service capacity of these establishments needs to be improved, especially for those in the Central and Western regions. The construction and service quality of small and medium-sized blood centers are unsatisfying. There is room for optimization of the function positioning of blood centers at various levels. The capacity to guarantee blood safety of primary blood collection and supply institutions is facing challenges.

II. The incentives for blood establishment employees needs to be improved.

The incentive measures for employees in blood centers need to be improved urgently, and the loss of some employees in blood centers has affected the normal operation of blood collection and supply. There is the lack of appropriate performance evaluation structure in blood collection and supply institutions. In some areas, the workload is not in line with and even divorced from the performance, resulting in poor economic incentives. There is no obvious distinction between the performance pay of the front-line personnel in blood collection and supply and highly professional and technical personnel and other employees, which dents the initiative of employees who do jobs with emergent, demanding, dangerous, severe, and highly technical content. Since available positions at public institutions are limited, it is common to offer low salaries to employees of the high-level positions, which, to some extents, affects and restricts the initiative of blood collection and supply practitioners.

III. The blood safety disciplines and professionals were underdeveloped.

Compared with developed countries, the development of blood transfusion medicine in China is inadequate. At present, there is no higher education training for blood transfusion medicine or blood safety related specialty in China. Most of the blood practitioners used to be in other clinical majors. In addition, there is no systematic continuing education for professionals. Blood transfusion medicine is an interdisciplinary subject. Compared with developed countries, China was not a late starter in blood transfusion medicine. However, the current development is slow, with distinct gaps from developed countries. This is not commensurate with the current social and economic development of China and the rapid development of other clinical specialties of medicine. This, to some extent, has affected safe supply and transfusion of blood in clinical settings.

IV. The capability for hemovigilance needs to be strengthened.

Hemovigilance platforms improve blood transfusion technology and blood safety management by monitoring adverse events related to blood transfusion (donation), analyzing the causes, and working out solutions and preventive measures. This has been the most widely adopted blood safety measure in developed countries, such as the United States and the United Kingdom. It has been recommended as the most effective and economical counter measure by the World Health Organization since the blood safety incident in France. At present, China has not established a national early intervention and early warning system on blood safety, which needs to be addressed. China's current laws and regulations lack clear support for the establishment of the early warning system for blood safety. The data-based risk and cause analyses and policy suggestions have not yet been formed. The scientific basis for government departments to formulate policies regarding blood transfusion and blood safety needs to be strengthened.

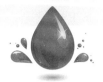

Chapter Three   Future Prospects

I. Stronger promotion of non-remunerated blood donation

Non-remunerated blood donation is a medical and health undertaking that serves the entire society. Local governments at different levels need to improve their long-term mechanism of non-remunerated blood donation with government leadership, inter-departmental cooperation, and public participation, create a supportive social climate for non-remunerated blood donation, give full play to advantages of the Red Cross Society of China and other non-governmental organizations, and encourage voluntary non-remunerated blood donation in the Party and government organs, enterprises, public institutions, universities and colleges, and communities. By expanding the base of non-remunerated blood donors and volunteers, the coordinated development of individual and group voluntary non-remunerated blood donation will be bolstered to facilitate safe and adequate supply of blood.

II. Better blood management information systems

China will strengthen the information-based blood management in an all-round way to realize the whole chain of blood informatization management from blood donors to blood users. It will gradually promote the network operation and information exchange of blood centers, plasma centers, medical institutions, disease control centers and other relevant departments to effectively screen high-risk blood donors, popularize electronic certificates of non-remunerated blood donation, comprehensively promote the online procedure of clinical blood exemptions, etc., realize the whole process information-based management of blood, so as to improve the blood supply support services.

III. More risk management capacity for blood safety

China will strengthen the risk management of blood safety, promote the monitoring of blood transfusion (donation) adverse reactions, and establish the mechanism of blood safety risk evaluation, assessment, decision-making, and prevention and control. By enhancing the all-rounded quality management of blood collection and supply institutions, China will improve the blood quality management ability of blood collection and supply institutions. It will also promote research on blood screening technology and strategies to improve the capability to detect pathogens transmitted by blood transfusion. The integrated guarantee mechanism of blood will be rolled out to achieve the balance between blood supply and demand. China will phase out targeted evaluation of rational use of blood at medical institutions to improve the clinical use of blood risk control.

IV. Innovative training for blood safety professionals

China will promote the training of blood safety professionals. by setting up the effective specialized curriculum system with the clear training direction to cultivate various levels of comprehensive blood safety professionals. It will strengthen the training of blood safety related expertise and regulations and improve skills of professionals. On-job, pre-job, and continuing education for blood center employees will be continued and enhanced.

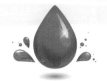

Appendices

Appendix 1   Summary of blood donation rates per 1,000 population in 2019

No.	Area	Blood donation rates per 1,000 population / per 1,000 population	Year on year	
			Growth/per 1,000 population)	Rate /%
1	Beijing	18.7	2.4	14.9
2	Tianjin	12.7	0.5	4.4
3	Hebei	11.2	0.6	5.6
4	Shanxi	10.6	0.7	7.5
5	Nei Mongol	8.6	−0.1	−0.9
6	Liaoning	9.7	−0.1	−1.2
7	Jilin	10.5	0.6	6.5
8	Heilongjiang	10.8	0.8	8.5
9	Shanghai	14.9	0.0	0.1
10	Jiangsu	13.7	0.7	5.7
11	Zhejiang	13.1	0.7	5.5
12	Anhui	8.3	0.5	6.0
13	Fujian	9.1	0.4	4.3
14	Jiangxi	9.1	0.5	6.3
15	Shandong	10.8	0.5	4.5

Continued

No.	Area	Blood donation rates per 1,000 population / per 1,000 population	Year on year	
			Growth/per 1,000 population)	Rate /%
16	Henan	12.7	0.4	3.3
17	Hubei	11.9	0.2	2.1
18	Hunan	9.0	0.4	4.4
19	Guangdong	12.7	0.7	5.6
20	Guangxi	11.9	0.7	6.5
21	Hainan	12.3	1.0	8.7
22	Chongqing	11.5	0.5	4.3
23	Sichuan	10.0	0.8	8.5
24	Guizhou	10.8	0.6	5.4
25	Yunnan	11.0	0.8	8.2
26	Xizang	1.3	0.9	188.5
27	Shaanxi	13.0	0.7	5.6
28	Gansu	8.2	0.1	1.1
29	Qinghai	8.0	0.3	4.6
30	Ningxia	9.8	0.4	4.0
31	Xinjiang	6.8	0.5	7.3
32	Corps	5.3	−0.6	−9.9

Appendix 2   Summary of the volume of blood donations in 2019

No.	Area	Whole blood			Platelet		
		Whole blood / KU	Year on year		Platelet / KTU	Year on year	
			Growth/ KU	Rate/ %		Growth/ KTU	Rate/ %
1	Beijing	559	53	10.5	112	24	26.8
2	Tianjin	372	83	28.8	60	5	9.0
3	Hebei	1,444	79	5.8	122	14	12.7
4	Shanxi	700	46	7.0	51	11	26.9
5	Nei Mongol	359	−0.4	−1.2	22	1	7.1

Continued

No.	Area	Whole blood			Platelet		
		Whole blood / KU	Year on year		Platelet / KTU	Year on year	
			Growth/ KU	Rate/ %		Growth/ KTU	Rate/ %
6	Liaoning	688	−18	−2.6	52	−1	−1.5
7	Jilin	456	32	7.4	30	2	8.2
8	Heilongjiang	688	51	8.0	36	−1	−1.6
9	Shanghai	463	6	1.3	49	3	7.6
10	Jiangsu	1,636	108	7.1	186	22	13.1
11	Zhejiang	1,077	74	7.4	142	46	47.4
12	Anhui	808	44	5.8	43	5	14.6
13	Fujian	552	23	4.3	39	2	5.3
14	Jiangxi	680	42	6.6	51	8	19.0
15	Shandong	1,751	84	5.0	141	13	10.2
16	Henan	2,178	71	3.4	173	15	9.3
17	Hubei	1,051	14	1.4	119	15	14.7
18	Hunan	1,033	53	5.5	77	9	13.9
19	Guangdong	2,104	124	6.3	193	35	22.4
20	Guangxi	945	56	6.3	54	7	14.9
21	Hainan	176	14	8.9	13	2	14.9
22	Chongqing	538	19	3.7	30	1	3.6
23	Sichuan	1,338	98	7.9	60	10	19.4
24	Guizhou	591	27	4.9	32	5	17.5
25	Yunnan	793	69	9.5	45	9	26.3
26	Xizang	5	4	210.6	0	0	—
27	Shaanxi	814	48	6.3	50	7	16.5
28	Gansu	315	6	2.0	16	2	15.1
29	Qinghai	84	3	3.7	22	−5	−17.6
30	Ningxia	122	5	4.7	6	1	10.8
31	Xinjiang	262	18	7.3	29	8	37.8
32	Corps	26	−2	−7.2	1	0	33.3

TU: Treatment Unit

Appendix 3   Summary of individual blood donation rates in 2019

No.	Area	Rate/%	Year on year	
			Growth/Percentage points	Rate/%
1	Beijing	70.3	0.0	−0.1
2	Tianjin	81.9	−3.2	−3.7
3	Hebei	81.0	2.6	3.3
4	Shanxi	78.6	−1.7	−2.1
5	Nei Mongol	83.5	−1.7	−2.0
6	Liaoning	73.8	−3.3	−4.3
7	Jilin	70.3	−0.3	−0.5
8	Heilongjiang	82.0	−1.0	−1.2
9	Shanghai	36.6	1.0	2.9
10	Jiangsu	65.1	1.0	1.6
11	Zhejiang	50.2	−1.6	−3.1
12	Anhui	81.9	3.2	4.1
13	Fujian	56.1	−4.4	−7.3
14	Jiangxi	65.8	−0.1	−0.2
15	Shandong	80.1	−0.5	−0.6
16	Henan	71.9	−11.2	−13.5
17	Hubei	87.4	−0.2	−0.2
18	Hunan	72.5	0.7	1.0
19	Guangdong	62.4	3.2	5.5
20	Guangxi	72.5	−2.0	−2.7
21	Hainan	71.8	8.3	13.0
22	Chongqing	83.9	−0.5	−0.5
23	Sichuan	56.9	−5.9	−9.4
24	Guizhou	83.2	−0.3	−0.4
25	Yunnan	62.8	−1.9	−2.9
26	Xizang	64.3	19.9	44.7
27	Shaanxi	82.9	−1.4	−1.7
28	Gansu	74.7	4.1	5.8
29	Qinghai	83.3	−0.6	−0.8
30	Ningxia	76.3	−7.4	−8.9
31	Xinjiang	87.2	2.7	3.2
32	Corps	99.2	0.0	0.0

Appendix 4   Summary of 400ml blood donation rates in 2019

No.	Area	Rate/%	Year on year	
			Growth/Percentage point	Rate/%
1	Beijing	64.9	−2.9	−4.3
2	Tianjin	76.2	−2.7	−3.5
3	Hebei	80.6	−0.3	−0.4
4	Shanxi	90.3	0.4	0.4
5	Nei Mongol	66.7	−0.4	−0.7
6	Liaoning	73.3	−1.6	−2.2
7	Jilin	55.9	0.4	0.7
8	Heilongjiang	76.2	−4.7	−5.9
9	Shanghai	38.5	1.7	4.6
10	Jiangsu	41.7	3.1	8.0
11	Zhejiang	37.5	−0.4	−1.1
12	Anhui	49.0	−1.7	−3.3
13	Fujian	45.7	−3.3	−6.7
14	Jiangxi	56.7	−1.1	−2.0
15	Shandong	62.6	−0.4	−0.7
16	Henan	91.1	−1.5	−1.6
17	Hubei	47.2	−2.6	−5.2
18	Hunan	57.9	3.9	7.2
19	Guangdong	45.0	−0.2	−0.3
20	Guangxi	57.0	−2.5	−4.2
21	Hainan	42.9	−9.3	−17.8
22	Chongqing	52.4	−2.1	−3.9
23	Sichuan	46.6	−3.9	−7.7
24	Guizhou	55.1	−1.2	−2.1
25	Yunnan	36.9	2.2	6.4
26	Xizang	1.6	−3.6	−68.7
27	Shaanxi	67.2	−0.1	−0.2
28	Gansu	29.1	−4.2	−12.6
29	Qinghai	79.7	−1.3	−1.7
30	Ningxia	82.7	−0.4	−0.4
31	Xinjiang	39.8	−15.1	−27.5
32	Corps	34.8	−2.9	−7.6

Appendix 5   Summary of confidential blood withdrawal rates in 2019

No.	Area	Confidential blood withdrawal /per 10,000	Year on year	
			Growth/per 10,000	Rate/%
1	Beijing	1.01	0.13	14.74
2	Tianjin	0.45	−0.22	−33.23
3	Hebei	0.18	−0.05	−22.51
4	Shanxi	11.06	10.03	973.69
5	Nei Mongol	5.19	5.14	9,873.90
6	Liaoning	0.16	−4.98	−96.98
7	Jilin	0.23	0.19	518.37
8	Heilongjiang	0.12	−0.40	−76.41
9	Shanghai	0.57	0.11	23.76
10	Jiangsu	0.69	0.28	67.83
11	Zhejiang	0.66	0.34	105.25
12	Anhui	0.47	−13.07	−96.56
13	Fujian	1.23	0.64	108.76
14	Jiangxi	0.28	0.17	167.33
15	Shandong	0.04	−0.31	−87.20
16	Henan	0.08	0.00	−3.65
17	Hubei	0.55	−0.13	−18.65
18	Hunan	0.17	−0.11	−39.82
19	Guangdong	2.26	−0.29	−11.30
20	Guangxi	0.23	−21.63	−98.97
21	Hainan	0.00	0.00	—
22	Chongqing	7.28	6.80	1,432.25
23	Sichuan	0.80	0.31	63.34
24	Guizhou	0.46	−0.38	−45.12
25	Yunnan	0.74	0.47	179.98
26	Xizang	20.62	−2.84	−12.09
27	Shaanxi	0.07	0.02	40.38
28	Gansu	24.99	12.86	105.98
29	Qinghai	9.41	4.84	105.88
30	Ningxia	0.24	−3.18	−93.11
31	Xinjiang	0.00	−0.17	−100.00
32	Corps	0.55	0.03	6.35

Appendix 6　Summary of female blood donor rates in 2019

No.	Area	Rate/%	Year on year	
			Growth/Percentage point	Rate/%
1	Beijing	31.3	0.6	2.0
2	Tianjin	26.2	0.6	2.2
3	Hebei	33.8	0.4	1.3
4	Shanxi	29.8	−0.4	−1.2
5	Nei Mongol	34.9	0.1	0.3
6	Liaoning	39.5	−0.1	−0.2
7	Jilin	37.5	0.8	2.2
8	Heilongjiang	41.0	0.5	1.3
9	Shanghai	32.2	1.8	5.8
10	Jiangsu	40.1	0.6	1.6
11	Zhejiang	39.0	0.7	1.9
12	Anhui	40.5	0.2	0.4
13	Fujian	38.1	0.3	0.8
14	Jiangxi	39.5	0.5	1.3
15	Shandong	30.1	0.4	1.4
16	Henan	37.0	0.0	−0.1
17	Hubei	38.7	0.6	1.6
18	Hunan	39.8	0.2	0.6
19	Guangdong	32.2	0.6	2.0
20	Guangxi	35.3	0.5	1.4
21	Hainan	29.8	−1.0	−3.4
22	Chongqing	50.1	−0.5	−1.0
23	Sichuan	48.7	0.6	1.2
24	Guizhou	51.8	0.4	0.8
25	Yunnan	45.3	0.6	1.4
26	Xizang	26.8	1.1	4.3
27	Shaanxi	37.8	0.2	0.4
28	Gansu	32.4	1.3	4.2
29	Qinghai	32.8	−0.9	−2.8
30	Ningxia	36.8	0.3	0.8
31	Xinjiang	33.9	0.0	0.1
32	Corps	35.6	0.9	2.7

Appendix 7　Summary of blood donation rates aged 18-35 in 2019

No.	Area	Rate/%	Year on year	
			Growth/Percentage point	Rate/%
1	Beijing	64.3	−0.6	−0.9
2	Tianjin	70.6	0.1	0.1
3	Hebei	45.7	−0.4	−1.0
4	Shanxi	43.8	0.8	1.9
5	Nei Mongol	45.5	−0.3	−0.6
6	Liaoning	48.8	0.8	1.6
7	Jilin	51.9	1.6	3.2
8	Heilongjiang	42.2	1.2	3.1
9	Shanghai	72.8	−0.6	−0.8
10	Jiangsu	50.5	−0.4	−0.8
11	Zhejiang	53.3	−0.4	−0.7
12	Anhui	52.0	0.0	0.0
13	Fujian	52.5	0.3	0.5
14	Jiangxi	56.1	0.0	0.1
15	Shandong	52.3	−0.3	−0.6
16	Henan	40.6	0.5	1.2
17	Hubei	51.5	−1.4	−2.6
18	Hunan	55.2	0.6	1.2
19	Guangdong	63.1	−0.5	−0.8
20	Guangxi	55.4	1.7	3.2
21	Hainan	60.7	−2.4	−3.8
22	Chongqing	49.2	−0.4	−0.8
23	Sichuan	43.1	0.0	0.1
24	Guizhou	56.5	0.3	0.6
25	Yunnan	61.4	0.7	1.2
26	Xizang	78.1	9.3	13.6
27	Shaanxi	53.8	−0.2	−0.4
28	Gansu	57.9	−0.2	−0.3
29	Qinghai	47.0	1.0	2.1
30	Ningxia	57.1	1.8	3.3
31	Xinjiang	59.9	2.6	4.5
32	Corps	56.7	−0.2	−0.4

Appendix 8   Summary of blood donation rates with bachelor degree or above in 2019

No.	Area	Rate/%	Year on year	
			Growth/Percentage point	Rate/%
1	Beijing	38.4	3.8	10.8
2	Tianjin	25.9	2.9	12.4
3	Hebei	15.2	−0.1	−0.4
4	Shanxi	21.3	2.1	11.0
5	Nei Mongol	23.6	0.4	1.6
6	Liaoning	24.5	3.5	16.7
7	Jilin	27.8	3.6	14.9
8	Heilongjiang	22.3	1.1	5.1
9	Shanghai	26.2	2.8	11.9
10	Jiangsu	22.0	0.5	2.2
11	Zhejiang	20.3	−1.9	−8.7
12	Anhui	26.0	1.4	5.7
13	Fujian	32.3	3.1	10.7
14	Jiangxi	26.1	0.6	2.3
15	Shandong	20.8	1.0	4.9
16	Henan	15.1	1.4	10.1
17	Hubei	26.2	−0.8	−3.1
18	Hunan	28.7	−0.1	−0.5
19	Guangdong	18.7	−0.6	−3.0
20	Guangxi	20.0	1.7	9.3
21	Hainan	27.6	−1.1	−3.9
22	Chongqing	21.0	0.0	−0.1
23	Sichuan	17.9	0.7	4.2
24	Guizhou	15.7	−0.2	−1.3
25	Yunnan	26.0	1.8	7.2
26	Xizang	32.9	11.5	53.9
27	Shaanxi	22.6	1.0	4.6
28	Gansu	20.9	1.5	7.6
29	Qinghai	20.1	0.5	2.6
30	Ningxia	23.8	3.7	18.5
31	Xinjiang	22.4	2.6	12.9
32	Corps	26.4	0.1	0.3

Appendix 9   Summary of blood testing at blood centers in 2019

No.	Area	Testing number			Ineligible number			Ineligible rate	
		Testing number/ TPT	Year on year		Ineligible number / TPT	Year on year		Rate/ %	Year on year
			Growth/ TPT	Rate/ %		Growth/ TPT	Rate/ %		Rate/ %
1	Beijing	475	63	15.3	74	13	21.3	15.5	0.8
2	Tianjin	228	10	4.6	29	2	6.2	12.8	0.2
3	Hebei	946	49	5.4	115	11	10.8	12.1	0.6
4	Shanxi	447	27	6.4	60	−2	−2.8	13.5	−1.3
5	Nei Mongol	228	06	2.5	26	1	6.2	11.2	0.4
6	Liaoning	478	−110	−18.7	78	−1	−1.8	16.4	2.8
7	Jilin	314	16	5.4	33	1	4.5	10.5	−0.1
8	Heilongjiang	419	5	1.2	38	−6	−12.9	9.1	−1.5
9	Shanghai	357	78	27.8	39	−3	−6.4	10.8	−4.0
10	Jiangsu	1,198	81	7.2	94	−1	−0.7	7.8	−0.6
11	Zhejiang	861	50	6.1	123	16	15.0	14.2	1.1
12	Anhui	557	31	6.0	43	1	1.3	7.8	−0.4
13	Fujian	398	12	3.2	45	−11	−20.0	11.3	−3.3
14	Jiangxi	442	13	3.0	34	−4	−10.0	7.8	−1.1
15	Shandong	1,165	55	4.9	105	9	9.0	9.0	0.3
16	Henan	1,313	36	2.8	144	18	14.0	11.0	1.1
17	Hubei	691	−8	−1.2	43	2	4.2	6.3	0.3
18	Hunan	647	28	4.6	39	−4	−8.2	6.1	−0.9
19	Guangdong	1,586	114	7.8	196	14	7.6	12.3	0.0
20	Guangxi	642	31	5.0	69	7	11.2	10.8	0.6
21	Hainan	132	11	8.8	19	0	0.0	14.2	−1.2
22	Chongqing	409	21	5.3	56	0	−0.7	13.6	−0.8
23	Sichuan	857	5	0.6	105	0	−0.2	12.2	−0.1
24	Guizhou	419	24	6.0	44	6	14.9	10.5	0.8
25	Yunnan	565	17	3.1	65	−5	−7.7	11.5	−1.4
26	Xizang	5	2	77.4	1	0	−22.8	21.8	−28.3
27	Shaanxi	534	23	4.6	39	−4	−9.6	7.3	−1.2

Continued

No.	Area	Testing number			Ineligible number			Ineligible rate	
		Testing number/ TPT	Year on year		Ineligible number / TPT	Year on year		Rate/ %	Year on year
			Growth/ TPT	Rate/ %		Growth/ TPT	Rate/ %		Rate/ %
28	Gansu	269	44	19.3	19	−4	−18.4	6.9	−3.2
29	Qinghai	59	2	3.2	13	0	2.3	21.4	−0.2
30	Ningxia	79	5	7.1	14	3	23.0	17.8	2.3
31	Xinjiang	184	8	4.5	24	2	9.7	13.2	0.6
32	Corps	17	−3	−15.5	2	−1	−30.3	10.6	−2.2

TPT: Thousand Person-Time

Appendix 10   Summary of pre-donation blood screening in 2019

No.	Area	Screening number			Ineligible number			Ineligible rate	
		Screening number / TPT	Year on year		Ineligible number / TPT	Year on year		Rate/ %	Year on year
			Growth/ TPT	Rate/ %		Growth/ TPT	Rate/ %		Rate/%
1	Beijing	475	63	15.3	66	12	22.2	13.9	0.8
2	Tianjin	228	10	4.6	26	1	5.0	11.6	0.0
3	Hebei	946	49	5.4	103	10	11.0	10.9	0.5
4	Shanxi	447	27	6.4	51	−2	−4.2	11.4	−1.3
5	Nei Mongol	228	6	2.5	20	1	5.1	8.7	0.2
6	Liaoning	478	−110	−18.7	73	−1	−1.0	15.2	2.7
7	Jilin	314	16	5.4	29	1	4.3	9.1	−0.1
8	Heilongjiang	419	5	1.2	31	−6	−16.8	7.5	−1.6
9	Shanghai	357	78	27.8	23	−5	−17.4	6.5	−3.6
10	Jiangsu	1,198	81	7.2	80	−1	−1.1	6.7	−0.6
11	Zhejiang	861	50	6.1	112	16	16.1	13.0	1.1
12	Anhui	557	31	6.0	31	−1	−3.5	5.6	−0.6
13	Fujian	398	12	3.2	37	−11	−23.2	9.4	−3.2
14	Jiangxi	442	13	3.0	27	−4	−12.7	6.0	−1.1
15	Shandong	1,165	55	4.9	88	10	12.5	7.6	0.5
16	Henan	1,313	36	2.8	116	9	8.1	8.9	0.4

Continued

No.	Area	Screening number			Ineligible number			Ineligible rate	
		Screening number / TPT	Year on year		Ineligible number / TPT	Year on year		Rate/ %	Year on year
			Growth/ TPT	Rate/ %		Growth/ TPT	Rate/ %		Rate/%
17	Hubei	691	−8	−1.2	28	1	3.0	4.0	0.2
18	Hunan	647	28	4.6	26	−3	−9.7	4.1	−0.6
19	Guangdong	1,586	114	7.8	148	7	5.1	9.3	−0.2
20	Guangxi	642	31	5.0	55	6	12.3	8.6	0.6
21	Hainan	132	11	8.8	16	0	1.9	12.2	−0.8
22	Chongqing	409	21	5.3	47	0	−0.3	11.4	−0.6
23	Sichuan	857	5	0.6	72	−4	−5.8	8.4	−0.6
24	Guizhou	419	24	6.0	32	5	17.0	7.6	0.7
25	Yunnan	565	17	3.1	53	−6	−10.1	9.4	−1.4
26	Xizang	5	2	77.4	1	0	−25.5	20.1	−27.7
27	Shaanxi	534	23	4.6	29	−5	−15.0	5.5	−1.3
28	Gansu	269	44	19.3	14	−4	−23.9	5.3	−3.0
29	Qinghai	59	2	3.2	11	0	−0.3	18.9	−0.7
30	Ningxia	79	5	7.1	13	3	23.7	16.8	2.3
31	Xinjiang	184	8	4.5	20	2	10.9	11.1	0.6
32	Corps	17	−3	−15.5	1	−1	−37.2	7.4	−2.5

TPT: Thousand Person-Time

Appendix 11　Summary of blood laboratory testing at blood centers in 2019

No.	Area	Testing number			Ineligible number			Ineligible rate	
		Testing number/ K	Year on year		Ineligible number/ K	Year on year		Rate/ %	Year on year
			Growth/ K	Rate/ %		Growth/ K	Rate/ %		Rate/%
1	Beijing	419	54	14.8	8	1	14.3	1.9	0.0
2	Tianjin	198	9	4.8	3	0	19.8	1.4	0.2
3	Hebei	853	54	6.7	11	1	9.3	1.3	0.0
4	Shanxi	406	28	7.5	9	1	6.2	2.2	0.0
5	Nei Mongol	229	0	−0.2	6	1	10.3	2.5	0.2

Continued

No.	Area	Testing number			Ineligible number			Ineligible rate	
		Testing number/ K	Year on year		Ineligible number/ K	Year on year		Rate/ %	Year on year
			Growth/ K	Rate/ %		Growth/ K	Rate/ %		Rate/%
6	Liaoning	430	3	0.8	6	−1	−10.3	1.3	−0.2
7	Jilin	290	22	8.0	4	0	6.3	1.5	0.0
8	Heilongjiang	410	30	8.0	7	1	12.4	1.6	0.1
9	Shanghai	351	3	0.8	15	2	17.0	4.4	0.6
10	Jiangsu	1,148	101	9.7	14	0	1.8	1.2	−0.1
11	Zhejiang	759	48	6.8	10	0	4.3	1.4	0.0
12	Anhui	529	32	6.4	12	2	16.3	2.3	0.2
13	Fujian	359	16	4.5	8	0	−0.7	2.2	−0.1
14	Jiangxi	418	22	5.6	8	0	1.0	1.9	−0.1
15	Shandong	1,094	54	5.2	17	−1	−6.2	1.6	−0.2
16	Henan	1,780	569	46.9	28	9	47.5	1.6	0.0
17	Hubei	711	−8	−1.1	15	1	6.5	2.1	0.2
18	Hunan	622	26	4.4	13	−1	−5.2	2.1	−0.2
19	Guangdong	1,536	126	8.9	48	7	16.0	3.1	0.2
20	Guangxi	632	31	5.1	14	1	7.0	2.2	0.0
21	Hainan	115	9	8.7	3	0	−10.1	2.3	−0.5
22	Chongqing	363	21	6.0	9	0	−2.9	2.5	−0.2
23	Sichuan	839	70	9.1	33	4	14.9	3.9	0.2
24	Guizhou	423	26	6.4	12	1	9.7	2.9	0.1
25	Yunnan	529	43	8.9	12	1	5.2	2.2	−0.1
26	Xizang	5	3	203.9	0	0	30.9	2.0	−2.6
27	Shaanxi	503	28	5.9	10	1	11.7	1.9	0.1
28	Gansu	216	3	1.4	4	0	7.0	2.0	0.1
29	Qinghai	50	2	4.6	1	0	27.6	2.9	0.5
30	Ningxia	68	3	5.2	1	0	13.0	1.1	0.1
31	Xinjiang	173	−7	−3.8	4	0	3.6	2.2	0.2
32	Corps	15	−2	−13.7	1	0	−6.9	3.5	0.3

Appendix 12　Summary of blood component separation rates in 2019

No.	Area	Rate/%	Year on year	
			Growth/Percentage point	Rate /%
1	Beijing	100.00	0.00	0.00
2	Tianjin	99.96	0.14	0.14
3	Hebei	99.83	0.13	0.13
4	Shanxi	99.26	−0.46	−0.46
5	Nei Mongol	99.81	0.49	0.49
6	Liaoning	99.87	0.01	0.01
7	Jilin	99.89	0.02	0.02
8	Heilongjiang	99.44	0.41	0.41
9	Shanghai	99.88	0.02	0.02
10	Jiangsu	99.98	0.01	0.01
11	Zhejiang	99.92	0.04	0.04
12	Anhui	99.91	0.05	0.05
13	Fujian	100.00	0.03	0.03
14	Jiangxi	100.00	0.00	0.00
15	Shandong	99.94	0.04	0.04
16	Henan	99.83	0.01	0.01
17	Hubei	99.95	0.01	0.01
18	Hunan	100.00	0.00	0.00
19	Guangdong	99.86	−0.12	−0.12
20	Guangxi	99.84	−0.14	−0.14
21	Hainan	99.98	−0.02	−0.02
22	Chongqing	99.94	0.27	0.27
23	Sichuan	99.98	0.00	0.00
24	Guizhou	99.96	0.01	0.01
25	Yunnan	100.00	0.00	0.00
26	Xizang	93.42	−4.44	−4.54

Continued

No.	Area	Rate/%	Year on year	
			Growth/Percentage point	Rate /%
27	Shaanxi	99.94	0.03	0.03
28	Gansu	99.85	0.09	0.09
29	Qinghai	98.47	−1.13	−1.13
30	Ningxia	99.97	2.75	2.82
31	Xinjiang	99.62	2.81	2.91
32	Corps	99.63	1.94	1.98

Appendix 13　Summary of platelet concentrate separation rates in 2019

No.	Area	Rate/%	Year on year	
			Growth/Percentage point	Rate/%
1	Beijing	0.5	−5.7	−91.4
2	Tianjin	12.1	1.5	13.8
3	Hebei	0.2	0.0	2.2
4	Shanxi	0.6	−0.1	−16.5
5	Nei Mongol	6.4	−2.1	−24.3
6	Liaoning	0.1	0.1	—
7	Jilin	0.5	−0.4	−42.6
8	Heilongjiang	0.3	0.1	54.0
9	Shanghai	1.5	0.6	61.1
10	Jiangsu	0.3	0.1	57.5
11	Zhejiang	0.2	−0.1	−31.2
12	Anhui	4.3	−0.8	−15.1
13	Fujian	4.5	3.5	346.5
14	Jiangxi	1.7	1.1	205.1
15	Shandong	0.0	0.0	73.1
16	Henan	0.5	0.3	134.7

Continued

No.	Area	Rate/%	Year on year	
			Growth/Percentage point	Rate/%
17	Hubei	0.0	−0.1	−100.0
18	Hunan	9.8	0.7	7.2
19	Guangdong	3.8	−3.9	−50.3
20	Guangxi	2.6	0.0	−0.8
21	Hainan	0.0	0.0	—
22	Chongqing	0.2	0.1	232.4
23	Sichuan	6.5	−0.6	−7.9
24	Guizhou	0.8	−0.2	−21.1
25	Yunnan	0.0	0.0	−100.0
26	Xizang	0.0	0.0	—
27	Shaanxi	1.1	−0.1	−8.4
28	Gansu	0.0	0.0	−74.5
29	Qinghai	3.1	−3.3	−51.6
30	Ningxia	17.7	16.9	2,234.2
31	Xinjiang	0.2	−0.3	−67.2
32	Corps	0.6	0.5	690.8

Appendix 14 Summary of total blood supply volume in 2019

No.	Area	Total blood supply volume /KU	Year on year	
			Growth/KU	Rate/%
1	Beijing	1,385	104	8.2
2	Tianjin	687	26	3.9
3	Hebei	2,754	243	9.7
4	Shanxi	1,189	127	11.9
5	Nei Mongol	631	−26	−4.0
6	Liaoning	1,351	80	6.3
7	Jilin	925	137	17.4

Continued

No.	Area	Total blood supply volume /KU	Year on year	
			Growth/KU	Rate/%
8	Heilongjiang	1,257	30	2.5
9	Shanghai	1,027	127	14.2
10	Jiangsu	3,768	643	20.6
11	Zhejiang	2,483	252	11.3
12	Anhui	1,558	137	9.6
13	Fujian	1,210	239	24.6
14	Jiangxi	1,564	315	25.2
15	Shandong	3,527	409	13.1
16	Henan	4,508	435	10.7
17	Hubei	2,174	228	11.7
18	Hunan	2,273	202	9.8
19	Guangdong	4,870	411	9.2
20	Guangxi	2,005	355	21.5
21	Hainan	367	88	31.6
22	Chongqing	1,115	117	11.7
23	Sichuan	2,316	230	11.0
24	Guizhou	1,130	108	10.6
25	Yunnan	1,613	256	18.9
26	Xizang	29	19	194.4
27	Shaanxi	1,662	201	13.7
28	Gansu	717	−659	−47.9
29	Qinghai	195	9	4.7
30	Ningxia	252	29	12.9
31	Xinjiang	668	150	28.9
32	Corps	55	−29	−34.4

Appendix 15　Summary of per capita blood consumption in 2019

No.	Area	Per capita blood consumption /ml	Year on year	
			Growth/ml	Rate/%
1	Beijing	5.8	0.4	6.9
2	Tianjin	3.7	0.1	2.6
3	Hebei	3.7	0.2	4.7
4	Shanxi	3.7	0.3	8.3
5	Nei Mongol	2.9	0.1	2.6
6	Liaoning	3.1	−0.1	−1.6
7	Jilin	3.3	0.3	10.9
8	Heilongjiang	3.6	0.3	10.3
9	Shanghai	3.6	0.1	3.7
10	Jiangsu	4.2	0.5	12.8
11	Zhejiang	3.6	0.2	5.6
12	Anhui	2.5	0.1	5.5
13	Fujian	3.0	0.4	14.4
14	Jiangxi	2.9	0.2	7.9
15	Shandong	3.4	0.1	3.8
16	Henan	4.5	0.2	3.8
17	Hubei	3.5	0.1	2.4
18	Hunan	2.9	0.2	6.4
19	Guangdong	4.0	0.7	20.6
20	Guangxi	3.8	0.3	9.8
21	Hainan	3.7	0.3	9.1
22	Chongqing	3.4	0.2	5.8
23	Sichuan	3.0	0.2	8.0
24	Guizhou	3.2	0.1	4.0

Continued

No.	Area	Per capita blood consumption /ml	Year on year	
			Growth/ml	Rate/%
25	Yunnan	3.3	0.3	10.0
26	Xizang	1.2	0.7	161.8
27	Shaanxi	4.1	0.2	5.0
28	Gansu	2.5	0.2	8.0
29	Qinghai	2.9	0.3	9.7
30	Ningxia	3.5	0.1	2.9
31	Xinjiang	2.1	0.1	6.6
32	Corps	1.8	0.0	−1.5

Appendix 16   Summary of platelet use volume (10,000 persons) in 2019

No.	Area	Use volume /TU	Year on year	
			Growth/TU	Rate/%
1	Beijing	63.115	10.904	20.9
2	Tianjin	40.668	3.528	9.5
3	Hebei	15.849	1.576	11.0
4	Shanxi	10.784	1.830	20.4
5	Nei Mongol	9.611	−0.970	−9.2
6	Liaoning	11.718	−0.304	−2.5
7	Jilin	11.121	0.900	8.8
8	Heilongjiang	9.790	0.066	0.7
9	Shanghai	23.105	3.454	17.6
10	Jiangsu	23.122	3.553	18.2
11	Zhejiang	19.147	1.910	11.1

Continued

No.	Area	Use volume /TU	Year on year	
			Growth/TU	Rate/%
12	Anhui	7.604	1.127	17.4
13	Fujian	11.085	1.564	16.4
14	Jiangxi	11.499	2.385	26.2
15	Shandong	14.000	1.271	10.0
16	Henan	18.102	1.494	9.0
17	Hubei	19.599	2.474	14.4
18	Hunan	12.519	1.541	14.0
19	Guangdong	18.251	3.079	20.3
20	Guangxi	11.172	1.206	12.1
21	Hainan	13.742	1.731	14.4
22	Chongqing	9.474	0.418	4.6
23	Sichuan	8.092	1.145	16.5
24	Guizhou	8.735	0.869	11.0
25	Yunnan	9.276	1.848	24.9
26	Xizang	0.109	0.109	—
27	Shaanxi	13.144	1.807	15.9
28	Gansu	5.734	0.659	13.0
29	Qinghai	36.135	−8.508	−19.1
30	Ningxia	11.305	3.543	45.6
31	Xinjiang	9.237	1.944	26.7
32	Corps	3.529	0.552	18.6

TU: Treatment Unit

Appendix 17　Summary of tangible components utilization rate in 2019

No.	Area	Rate/%	Year on year	
			Growth/Percentage point	Rate/%
1	Beijing	100.5	−5.7	−5.4
2	Tianjin	112.0	1.6	3.4
3	Hebei	100.0	0.1	0.3
4	Shanxi	99.9	−0.6	−1.0
5	Nei Mongol	106.2	−1.6	−2.7
6	Liaoning	100.0	0.1	0.3
7	Jilin	100.4	−0.4	−0.7
8	Heilongjiang	99.7	0.5	1.0
9	Shanghai	101.4	0.6	1.2
10	Jiangsu	100.3	0.1	0.2
11	Zhejiang	100.1	0.0	−0.1
12	Anhui	104.2	−0.7	−1.3
13	Fujian	104.5	3.5	6.5
14	Jiangxi	101.7	1.1	2.3
15	Shandong	100.0	0.1	0.1
16	Henan	100.3	0.3	0.6
17	Hubei	100.0	0.0	−0.1
18	Hunan	109.8	0.7	1.3
19	Guangdong	103.7	−4.0	−8.8
20	Guangxi	102.4	−0.2	−0.3
21	Hainan	100.0	0.0	0.0
22	Chongqing	100.1	0.4	0.7
23	Sichuan	106.5	−0.6	−0.9
24	Guizhou	100.7	−0.2	−0.3

Continued

No.	Area	Rate/%	Year on year	
			Growth/Percentage point	Rate/%
25	Yunnan	100.0	0.0	0.0
26	Xizang	93.4	−4.4	−5.9
27	Shaanxi	101.1	−0.1	−0.2
28	Gansu	99.9	0.1	0.3
29	Qinghai	101.6	−4.5	−9.9
30	Ningxia	117.7	19.7	38.9
31	Xinjiang	99.8	2.5	5.5
32	Corps	100.2	2.4	7.6